The *Living Well with Dementia* Course

The Living Well with Dementia *Course: A Workbook for Facilitators* will be an indispensable guide to providing support to people after they have received a dementia diagnosis. The workbook provides facilitators with a realistic but positive approach to helping people with dementia understand and adjust to their condition, helping them to live as well as possible.

This workbook outlines the *Living Well with Dementia* course, a post-diagnostic course for people who have recently received a diagnosis of dementia. Its session-by-session structure, along with e-resources including handouts for course participants, will help facilitators provide a realistic but positive approach to support after a diagnosis.

Aimed at facilitators, and drawing on the authors' many years of clinical and research experience, *The* Living Well with Dementia *Course* workbook will be of great assistance to healthcare professionals and support workers in many different settings, including specialist NHS dementia services, primary care services and the voluntary and community sector.

Richard Cheston is Professor of Dementia Research at the University of the West of England. Between 1998 and 2012, he worked as a Consultant Clinical Psychologist with Avon and Wilts NHS Partnership Trust. He is also an Honorary Senior Research Fellow, RICE Memory Clinic.

Ann Marshall is Consultant Clinical Psychologist. She qualified at the Institute of Psychiatry, London in 1981 and between 1988 and 2018 worked in NHS Older People's Mental Health services in Hampshire and as an honorary tutor at Southampton University.

"This book is so much more than a workbook for running a course! 'Living Well with Dementia' is a phrase that has become very over-used in recent years. Whilst it is a great aim, many people struggle with how to achieve living well on a practical level. Richard Cheston and Ann Marshall have been helping people to adjust to the changes that dementia brings for many years. It is full of their wisdom. It will be a go-to resource for those with lots of knowledge about dementia but who feel less sure about how to use counselling skills to help people adjust emotionally. Likewise, it will be very helpful to those who may feel confident in their counselling skills but who do not know how to apply these to support those living with dementia. I highly recommend this book."

Professor Dawn Brooker, Director of the Association for Dementia Studies, University of Worcester

"I wholeheartedly commend this comprehensive guide to those seeking to deliver or draw extra benefit from this *Living Well with Dementia* course. As someone who has tried to live well with dementia for eight years, I know how beneficial it would have been to me. After diagnosis, my wife and I attended two afternoons designed to lead us away from the 'cliff edge' to which I was clinging; I am totally convinced that this would have been far more successful had this excellent guide been available at that time."

Keith Oliver, Alzheimer's Society Ambassador and 3 Nations Dementia Working Group

"The emotional impact of developing dementia is immense, and without support many people struggle to adjust. The *Living Well with Dementia* course is unique in its focus on enabling people with dementia to reflect and share their experiences and find a way to talk about and accept what is happening. In this accessible guide, Rik Cheston and Ann Marshall provide a session-by-session outline for course facilitators, supported by in-session activities and handouts, practical tips on how to plan, prepare and run the course, and advice on training and supervision. This is a 'must read' for anyone involved in supporting people living with mild to moderate dementia."

Professor Linda Clare, University of Exeter

The *Living Well with* Dementia Course

- A Workbook for Facilitators

Richard Cheston and Ann Marshall

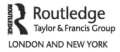
Routledge
Taylor & Francis Group

LONDON AND NEW YORK

First published 2019
by Routledge
2 Park Square, Milton Park, Abingdon, Oxon OX14 4RN

and by Routledge
52 Vanderbilt Avenue, New York, NY 10017

Routledge is an imprint of the Taylor & Francis Group, an informa business

Illustrations by Will Mower

British Library Cataloguing-in-Publication Data
A catalogue record for this book is available from the British Library

Library of Congress Cataloging-in-Publication Data
Names: Cheston, Richard, 1961– author.
Title: The living well with dementia course : a workbook for facilitators / Richard Cheston and Ann Marshall.
Description: Milton Park, Abingdon, Oxon ; New York, NY : Routledge, 2019. | Includes bibliographical references and index.
Identifiers: LCCN 2019001324 (print) | LCCN 2019001657 (ebook) | ISBN 9781351009003 (Master E-Book) | ISBN 9781138542341 (hardback : alk. paper) | ISBN 9781138542358 (pbk. : alk. paper) | ISBN 9781351009003 (ebk)
Subjects: LCSH: Dementia. | Self-help techniques—Study and teaching.
Classification: LCC RC521 (ebook) | LCC RC521 .C44 2019 (print) | DDC 616.8/31—dc23
LC record available at https://lccn.loc.gov/2019001324

ISBN: 978-1-138-54234-1 (hbk)
ISBN: 978-1-138-54235-8 (pbk)
ISBN: 978-1-351-00900-3 (ebk)

Typeset in Stone Serif
by Apex CoVantage, LLC

Printed and bound by CPI Group (UK) Ltd, Croydon, CR0 4YY
Visit the eResources: www.routledge.com/9781138542358

We'd like to dedicate this book to the many people living with dementia and their families who have worked with us over the years.

Contents

Preface

The origins of this workbook are somewhat accidental, as both of us somewhat stumbled into running our first groups. For Ann, the initial impetus came after a doctor in her memory clinic realised that a trend towards earlier dementia diagnosis (partly prompted by the new cholinesterase inhibitor medication available) meant that they were increasingly seeing people at an earlier stage in the illness. She suggested establishing a group to teach patients useful coping strategies. For Rik, the drive to run a group came after being given the chance to take up a place in a training course on Validation Therapy that a colleague could no longer attend.

From an early point, however, running these groups meant that both of us began to ask questions about what we were doing: we each began to realise that the participants in our group were much keener to explore how others in the group were coping from an emotional perspective rather than just learn new memory strategies. They also wanted to make sense out of what was happening to them, their identity and relationships as well as finding new meaning and purpose, often with a desire to help others in a similar situation.

At that stage, during the mid-1990s, support groups for people who were living with dementia were something of a rarity. Post-diagnostic educational and support groups for carers were relatively common, but there was a widespread assumption that people who had dementia were either not capable of benefitting from this sort of intervention or that to try and talk about the dementia might simply make them even more upset. Many of those health care professionals whose job it was to assess and to make a diagnosis of dementia or to provide support after this did not, therefore, routinely talk to the people they were working with about what was happening to them. That's not to say that they didn't talk to people with dementia – they did, for instance, by reminiscing about their life, or by talking about specific ways of remembering things. What was missing, however, was having a conversation about the diagnosis. Where health care workers did have these sorts of dialogue, then all too often they tended to be with the person's relatives.

Now, thankfully, people working in memory clinics and voluntary groups increasingly see the need for a place where people can talk about their diagnosis and learn about how to make the most out of their lives. However, wanting to help people to discuss this difficult subject and knowing how to start doing so are two separate things – and this is the gap that this workbook sets out to fill. In writing this workbook, we realise that talking to people about their dementia is rarely, if ever, a simple process. We also appreciate that not everyone who has dementia wants to, or needs to, talk about the illness. In many cases, people go to great lengths *not* to talk about what is happening – and trying to do so may be precisely the wrong thing to do.

What we do believe, however, is that talking to people about what they're going through and what is to come is often just as important for someone with dementia as it is for a person who has a diagnosis of cancer or any other serious illness. Unless people living with dementia have these conversations, it will be much harder for them to accept the illness, to prepare for the future and to make the most of the present. Without talking about what is happening, it will be so much harder to live well with dementia. It is so much easier to learn that you're not alone, and that you can live with your dementia, if you meet other people who are trying to do the same thing.

With our best wishes for the conversations that lie ahead of you!

Acknowledgements

We would like to recognise the debt we owe our many colleagues, friends, students and trainees over the past years. This includes the many people who have contributed to the development of the *Living Well with Dementia* course over the years: Peter Coleman, John Spreadbury, Clive Holmes, Elizabeth Bartlett and Liz Howells, as well as the many course facilitators in Wiltshire and Hampshire who led our first groups and took part in our research. There are many other colleagues whose support in developing this workbook over the years has been so important – too numerous to list separately, so we will list them here alphabetically to convey our gratitude: Jeremy Allen, Gillian Bebber, Nick Bennians, Stephany Bowen, Romola Bucks, David Childs, Peter Clegg, Lorraine Conduit, Suzanne Davis, Elizabeth Drew, Jane Fossey, Julia Gifford, Rebecca Guhan, Julia Hecquet, Lynne Hopkinson, Julian Hughes, Zoe Hughes, Ada Ivanecka, Charlie Jones, Roy Jones, Jo Keightley, Anna Littlechild, Helen Mander, Jill Mann, Chris Pawson, Gill Podger, Shanté Richardson, Elsa Schmidt, Debbie Smith, John Spreadbury, Deirdre Sutton-Smith, Paul Whitby, Philippa Wilson, Liz Young and Nancy Zook. Additionally, our clinical work has been supported and developed by working with so many excellent local clinicians within the community Mental Health Teams in Avon and Wiltshire Mental Health Partnership Trust, Southern Health Partnership and at the RICE Memory Clinic in Bath.

The *Living Well with Dementia* course has also benefited enormously from the feedback we have had from clinicians in the UK and Ireland who have been using previous versions of the workbook: Deborah Becker, Alexis Berry, John Burns, Kim Henderson, Tina Lee, Tracey Lintern, Alice Loyal, Rosslyn Offord, Jane Pritchard, Rebecca Read, Lawrence Wintergold and Naomi Wynne-Morgan.

We would also like to recognise the organisations that have funded different aspects of this research that we report here: the Mental Health Foundation, the National Institute for Health Research (NIHR), the Alzheimer's Society, Alzheimer's Research UK and the University of the West of England. The views expressed here are ours, and ours alone, and do not reflect the views of any of these agencies.

We would also like to acknowledge our gratitude to the many Clinical Psychology trainees and assistants who we have been fortunate to learn from and to be challenged by over our careers.

Above all, we'd like to thank the many people with dementia, their families and friends we have known and worked with. Without their willingness to share their experiences, we could not have begun to write this book, and we hope that they feel we have been able to communicate some of that learning here.

Finally, we are both indebted to the support, patience and tolerance of our families over the past years: Andrea, Katharine, Huw, Derek, Tim, Dominic and Lucy.

1 Introduction to the *Living Well with Dementia* course

There are around 850,000 people who are living with dementia in the UK. All of the national governments within the UK now place great emphasis on making sure that people with dementia are diagnosed at as early a point as possible. Increasingly, the National Health Service (NHS) and other services also make sure that information and support are available after a diagnosis. This aim of this support is to provide the opportunity for people to adjust to the illness better and to develop new coping skills.

In the UK, there are many different forms of support currently available – sometimes a confusingly large number of therapies, supports and advisors, including Animal-Assisted Therapy, Assistive Technology, Cognitive Behavioural Therapy, Cognitive Rehabilitation, Cognitive Stimulation Therapy, Creative Arts Therapies, Dementia Advisors and Navigators, Alzheimer Cafés, Singing for the Brain, Life Review Therapy, Life Story Work, Music Therapy and Reminiscence Therapy, to name just a few. However, while all of these different sources of support and therapy can be extremely useful, all too often the emotional impact of dementia is not addressed. In particular, the process by which people adjust to their diagnosis is all too often ignored. It is precisely this need that the *Living Well with Dementia* course focuses on – providing the support that many people who have recently been diagnosed with dementia need to help them to adjust to, accept and come to terms with their diagnosis.

The importance of emotional support

We believe that it is often the emotions that surround dementia that make it difficult for people to talk about it. People may be worried about the future, angry and frustrated at their memory loss or grieving for what is now beyond them. Often, it is difficult for their family and friends, who are themselves trying to adjust to the illness, to know how to provide the emotional support that is needed.

Providing emotional support can help people to talk more openly about their illness – and thus to adjust to their condition. However, emotional support needs to be provided at a pace that is appropriate for the person, either following diagnosis or when the person feels ready. Ideally, support should also be available to the person's family or other people closely involved – both to help them to adjust and to promote discussion between them as a couple or as a family.

It is important for people who have a diagnosis of dementia to have the opportunity to understand more about their illness if they wish to do so. However, this can be challenging: dementia is a frightening illness. For many people, a safe, supportive course with an experienced facilitator can enable people to meet others who are going through the same things as they are and take away some of the fear about dementia. The groups also provide a chance for people to learn from and to help each other.

Why is dementia difficult to discuss?

The vast majority of people who go to a memory clinic or consult their GP about their memory difficulties want to be told what is wrong with them – they want to be given their diagnosis, even if this is upsetting. However, once they leave the memory clinic, then often it can be difficult for them to find a way to continue to think and to talk about their diagnosis. There are very understandable reasons for this:

- **Receiving a diagnosis is frightening.** Dementia is a progressive illness that cannot be cured and which involves the person gradually losing many of the abilities that define him or her and becoming increasingly dependent on others. It's no wonder that people are frightened about what lies ahead. However, people often have misconceptions – for instance, thinking that they will rapidly deteriorate, or that they won't be able to have any quality of life.
- **Dementia and stigma.** We know that there is often a stigma about dementia. This is one of the most important barriers to talking about memory problems and something that often stops people receiving a diagnosis and the support that comes with this. One of the most common reactions to stigma is that people prefer not to talk about their problems. One *Living Well with Dementia* course participant said, *"You don't like to talk about it. I kept it to myself before I said anything, and wouldn't tell anyone. I thought that they'd think I was mad"*.

   There is evidence that people from some black, Asian and minority ethnic (BAME) communities may be especially vulnerable to feelings of shame following a diagnosis of dementia (1, 2). Within many BAME communities, the changes that memory services view as "symptoms" of dementia either seem to be just a feature of growing old or are seen as highly stigmatised signs of mental illness. In addition, sometimes families feel an especially intense pressure to provide care themselves without relying on support from the outside world. Consequently, the feelings of shame and embarrassment that are felt by almost everyone who is living with dementia tend to be intensified for many people from some BAME communities.

- *Other people might also avoid talking about dementia* with the person who has been diagnosed, not knowing how to approach it. As one man told us in a group:

  "People can't handle it so they don't want to know, so they try to avoid it".

- **People may feel embarrassed.** People often feel embarrassed about having a memory problem or other types of cognitive difficulties and tend to avoid situations where the problems might be exposed. This can lead to them feeling lonely and isolated, which can make their problems worse.

Due to all of these very understandable feelings, a common response of people who have received the diagnosis is to begin to withdraw into themselves. It is as if they have chosen, in some way, to "shut off" their awareness about their dementia – for instance, by withdrawing from activities and being reluctant to talk about their dementia. For some people, this shutting off of awareness may well be the best way to cope. However, this is not always the case – often it is important to provide people who have been recently diagnosed with opportunities to understand their illness and a space to think through its implications. We believe that providing these opportunities often enables people to cope better. This is exactly what we think this course can provide.

How does the *Living Well with Dementia* course help?

The approach in this course is that one of the best ways to help people to live well with dementia is to help them to find a way to talk about their experiences and difficulties. Often, people either avoid talking about their dementia or refer to it indirectly – as "it" or "that thing I've got". It can be a big step for people to use terms such as "dementia" or "Alzheimer's disease", because, for many people, this makes it more immediate and present in their lives. An important psychological task, then, is for people to not only name their illness, but also do so without being emotionally overwhelmed by its implications.

At the same time, it is important for those providing this support to realise that not everybody wants to talk about their dementia or is able to do this. This inability to talk openly about dementia may be due to many different factors – including the neurological impact of the illness itself. Sometimes, it may be because the person has always struggled to accept change. For some people, other ways of coping will be preferable, and the *Living Well with Dementia* course will not be for them.

In order to help people with the emotional elements of adjusting, the approach we have taken in this workbook is to be gentle and supportive and to find a way to help group members feel comfortable.

So use this workbook in the way that works best for your course. You will need to go at the pace that's right for the group members and which creates a space where they feel comfortable discussing difficult and emotional issues. However you use the workbook, there are some basic principles that you should follow to maximise the opportunity for people to "live well with their dementia".

Measuring effectiveness – what differences does coming to a *Living Well with Dementia* course make?

In the time that we have been using and developing the *Living Well with Dementia* course, we have made a conscious effort to continue a research programme to learn more about its clinical impact. This includes asking for feedback from all of the NHS services that have been using it. This feedback has been integrated into successive versions of the workbook and has helped us to continue to develop the model.

This research programme has combined quantitative research (such as comparing levels of self-esteem and quality of life before and after participants complete the course) and qualitative research (for instance, interviewing participants, their families and group leaders to find out their opinions). Sometimes this research has been specifically funded through a grant, and at other times group facilitators have asked people attending the course to complete an evaluation form at the end. In considering this evidence, it is important to bear two things in mind: first, we have not yet been able to carry out the detailed, extensive research that would conclusively demonstrate, one way or another, whether the *Living Well with Dementia* course is effective; second, while we believe that the evidence that we have so far collected does point to some people benefitting from the *Living Well with Dementia* course, at the same time, there are other people who clearly don't benefit. This may be because they attend all the way through the course but just don't feel that the course has helped them, or because they come to a few sessions and then decide it's not for them.

Participants feel better about themselves

Perhaps the most frequent comment that people who have come to a course make at the end is that they feel better and more confident about themselves. One participant on a Northampton course, for instance, said that it had given them *"the confidence to deal with the initial problems that the dementia is causing"*. As psychologists, we describe this as people having a higher level of self-esteem – something that dementia generally erodes. We know that good self-esteem is important for many reasons, including helping people to deal with change. It was, therefore, one of the main things we looked at in a pilot study of the *Living Well with Dementia* course (3). In this, we compared 30 people who were randomly allocated to attend a course and 30 people who were allocated to waiting to attend a course (a control group). This study was a pilot study – it wasn't intended to find definitive results, but rather help us to be confident of the methodology that we could use in a larger trial, including the process of randomisation, training facilitators, and so on. The results of this pilot study were mixed: attending the course did improve self-esteem, but once we took into account differences between the two groups at the start of the course, then this improvement wasn't statistically significant, probably because our sample was quite small.

However, the pilot study is not the only research into the course that has been carried out. Clinicians in two NHS sites (led by Alexis Berry in Northampton and Tracy Lintern in Sussex) have been running *Living Well with Dementia* courses for several years and have been collecting data from course participants as they have done so. These studies don't have the methodological advantages of including a control group, but they still provide important evidence about whether people change as a result of attending a course. Both of these studies have shown significant improvements in average levels of self-esteem as a result of attending the course: in Northamptonshire, this was the case for 128 participants and in Sussex, for 38 participants.

Participants often have a better quality of life

As people feel better about themselves, they also develop the confidence to face challenges in their life. One Northampton participant said, *"The group gave me time to think about how I would manage frustrations about forgetting things. I have learnt not to get narky with myself about it. I read more now and get books from the library"*. The same picture comes from Sussex, where one participant reported that *"I feel more confident and want to do more e.g. outings, simple chores"*, while another said, *"I am now doing more and reading more, going out instead of sitting at home watching TV"*.

Carers, too, often say that their partner has developed the confidence to do more things. One woman recognised this in her husband, who she said had *"gained more awareness of a shared experience with others which reduced his feelings of isolation and indifference"*. A carer in Northampton reported a similar experience: *"most importantly the group halted a decline into 'closing down' life, so life is opening up. We are looking at what is possible as opposed to what has been lost"*.

One way of measuring whether these anecdotal reports of participants doing more as a consequence of attending a course are isolated incidents or reflect a more general pattern of change is to assess whether the course improves participants' quality of life. In our pilot study, we found that average levels of quality of life improved for participants in the *Living Well with Dementia* course compared with those in the control group, but once again not to an extent to be statistically significant. However, the results from the *Living Well with Dementia* course in Northampton did show a significant improvement in quality of life for participants as well as a reduction in the extent to which carers felt stressed.

Participants are more able to accept their dementia

One of our main aims in developing the *Living Well with Dementia* course was to create a safe way for participants to discuss their dementia with other people who had similar experiences and who could, therefore, understand how they felt. For many people, this is exactly what has happened. In sharing their experiences, participants came to realise that they are not the only ones experiencing these symptoms. As a Sussex participant put it, *"I didn't realise there were others in the same situation as me. I felt quite alone before the group".* For many people, this apparently simple insight is an enormously important step. For instance, one man described how his wife *"now realises what has happened to her and is now taking this in her stride. She has enjoyed knowing that she will be amongst people with the same problems she has and being able to share and talk about her issues".*

In order for these changes in thinking about dementia to happen, it is important for participants to be able to talk openly about their lives with dementia. A woman who came to one of the courses in our pilot study told us at the end, *"I'm not ashamed to say that I've got it [dementia] whereas I think I might have been if it hadn't been, you know, for everybody else being so honest".* Her husband agreed with her, saying, *"Probably the most important thing, is it encouraged you in front of other people to stand up and say 'I have dementia'. . . . I think up until that hospital session she was in denial that she had it but after that she wasn't in denial and that helped a hell of a lot I think".* He added, *"Although [this] seems small it is very, very big. I mean once you've accepted you've got a problem then you will accept people trying to help you more. But if you're in denial that you have this problem then of course you're not prepared to accept help from anybody".*

In our pilot study, we wanted to see if there was any evidence for this change in how people talked about their dementia. To do this, we asked for permission from participants to record the groups – we then transcribed these recordings and analysed them by coding every time someone on the course refers to having dementia or acknowledges having a memory problem (4). We found that over the duration of the course, participants did tend to talk about their dementia in a different way. In the first few weeks, the main way in which participants talked was to refer to the dementia indirectly, for instance, as "it" or "that thing". Sometimes participants did not acknowledge having a problem at all, and at other times talked about having to fight a battle against an enemy perhaps by describing stories from their past. Typically, however, they don't refer openly and directly to their dementia even to the point of avoiding using the words "dementia" or "Alzheimer's disease". When they did refer to their dementia, they tended to do so in an unemotional way.

Over time, however, another way of talking emerged, with course participants being more able to reflect on how their dementia made them feel. Sometimes this was difficult for course facilitators and their fellow participants to hear, as there could be moving descriptions of feeling stuck or overwhelmed or fearful about the future. Occasionally, participants spoke of how starting to talk about their illness made them feel afraid that they were losing control in some way. However, despite their fears, for many people, beginning to share their difficult feelings was helpful – for instance, it enabled some people to feel that their worst fears can be confronted and that they were shared by others in the group. In other words, they realised that they were not alone with these feelings.

In the final sessions, however, a third way of talking emerged – participants began to be both emotional and practical. They were more likely to talk about learning new techniques and of feeling proud of coping in a different way. They could talk about dementia directly, and they no longer hid the diagnosis away; instead, they were being more open about it. One participant's feedback stated that *"it was tremendously valuable to meet people in similar circumstances and to share experiences. It was like a control mechanism to help release how you are feeling"*. Carers also noticed similar changes, with one reporting about her husband: *"The changes were that he shows his emotions now and he never did. The group brought him out of himself and now he talks about his feelings more"*. A second woman said of her husband, *"The group put him in a different frame of mind. He was depressed before he attended because he had dementia and now it's lightened it"*.

Talking to other people about dementia

One consequence for participants of being more able to accept their diagnosis is that many participants felt more able to talk to their family and friends about having dementia. This is a topic that sessions 5 and 6 explore in more detail – and while our approach is not to advise people that they should tell others but always to ask participants to think over the advantages and disadvantages of talking openly, this is clearly something that some participants feel more able to do as a consequence of coming to the course. Amongst the feedback we have had are comments such as *"I've been able to tell people about having dementia and been given the confidence to do that"*; *"I now tell people 'I have dementia'. . . . I haven't got a problem with it now"*; *"It wasn't until I came to the group that I realised – just tell them"*; and *"I now feel that the best thing to do is to tell friends that you have dementia and not be afraid of it"*.

How can we help people to talk about their dementia?

As well as looking at whether the language used by participants changes, we also have begun to look at how course facilitators can help participants to talk more openly about their dementia (4, 5, 6). We did this by comparing recordings of two courses that had been run by different pairs of facilitators in two different sessions: the first towards the start of the course (week two) and the second in the final session (week eight). For each session, we analysed both the language that participants used to describe their dementia and the ways in which the facilitators interacted with them. In week two, the way in which participants talked about their dementia in both courses was the same and was typical of the sort of thing we would expect: participants tended to talk in general and quite vague terms about their dementia, using the indirect language we have described earlier. In week eight, however, the way in which participants talked in the two courses was very different: in the first course, participants spoke very little about their dementia, and when they did so, the language they used was very similar to the language they used in week two. In effect, not only had there been no change in how they talked about their dementia, but also they actually spoke less about it. In the second course, however, dementia was described in a very different way, with the emotional impact of dementia being openly talked about and participants describing themselves as having changed and being less overwhelmed by the diagnosis.

So what had caused this difference between the two courses? Well, we can't know for sure – any experienced group worker will testify that some groups just don't gel. It may be, then, that no matter what the facilitators did, we would have found these differences. However, what emerged was that there was an important difference between the ways in which the course facilitators worked. In the second course, the facilitators tended to ask participants open rather than closed questions and used what counsellors call "reflection" – in effect, summarising what a participant has said. Both of these ways of facilitating tend to have the effect of encouraging people to say more. By contrast, the facilitators on the first course asked fewer questions and tended to give participants lots of information, including telling them what they should be thinking or saying. In effect, our analysis suggested that the facilitators on the first course tended to say more, and to listen rather less, to participants. Often, this is a sign of inexperienced, and possibly rather nervous, facilitators. By contrast, the facilitators on the second course seemed to be more relaxed and to feel more comfortable in allowing participants to explore their feelings.

> *It occurred to me that at one point it was like I had two diseases – one was Alzheimer's and the other was knowing that I had Alzheimer's.*
>
> *There were times when I thought I'd have been much happier not knowing, just accepting that I'd lost brain cells and one day they'd probably grow back or whatever. It is better to know, though, and better for it to be known.*
>
> *The first step is to talk openly about dementia because it's a fact, well enshrined in folklore, that if we are to kill the demon, then first we have to speak its name.*
>
> *Once we have recognised the demon, without secrecy or shame, we can find its weaknesses.*
>
> Terry Pratchett (*The Observer*, 15.03.15) (7)

References

1   Moriarty, J., Sharif, N. and Robinson, J. (2011) *Black and Minority Ethnic People with Dementia and Their Access to Support and Services.* London: Social Care Institute for Excellence.

2   APPG (All-Party Parliamentary Group) on Dementia (2013) *Dementia Does Not Discriminate: The Experience of Black, Asian and Minority Ethnic Communities.* London: Alzheimer's Society.

3   Marshall, A., Spreadbury, J., Cheston, R., Coleman, P., Ballinger, C., Mullee, M., Pritchard, J., Russell, C. and Bartlett, E. (2015) A Pilot Randomised Control Trial to Compare Changes in Quality of Life for Participants with Early Diagnosis Dementia Who Attend a "Living Well with Dementia" Group Compared to Waiting List Control, *Aging and Mental Health*, 19 (6), 526–535, doi: 10.1080/13607863.2014.954527.

4   Cheston, R., Gatting, L., Marshall, A., Spreadbury, J. and Coleman, P. (2017) Markers of Assimilation of Problematic Experiences in Dementia within the LIVDEM Project, *Dementia: The International Journal of Social Research and Policy*, 16 (4), 443–460, doi: 10.1177/1471301215602473.

5   Cheston, R., Marshall, A., Jones, A., Spreadbury, J. and Coleman, P. (2018) Living Well with Dementia Groups: Changes in Participant and Therapist Verbal Behaviour, *Aging and Mental Health*, 22 (1), 61–69, doi: 10.1080/13607863.2016.1231171.

6   Watkins, R., Cheston, R., Jones, K. and Gilliard, J. (2006) "Coming Out" with Alzheimer's Disease: Changes in Awareness during a Psychotherapy Group for People with Dementia, *Aging and Mental Health*, 10, 166–176.

7   Pratchett, T. (2015) You Can't Battle Alzheimer's . . . It Steals You from Yourself, *Guardian News & Media Limited*, 15 May.

2 Setting up and leading a *Living Well with Dementia* course

Principles in running a *Living Well with Dementia* course

If you have experience of working with people with dementia soon after diagnosis and also have some experience of working with groups, then you will probably feel comfortable in using the material in the guide to run a *Living Well with Dementia* course. We use the term "course" to describe *Living Well with Dementia* because we see it as providing opportunities to learn about and understand dementia. However, we also recognise that it is often the emotional aspects of adjusting to dementia that are the hardest, so it is important for group facilitators to feel comfortable working with often difficult emotions. In order to facilitate a *Living Well with Dementia* course, then, it is also important to have some basic ideas about working with emotions. Whether you have run something similar to this course before, there are some general points to bear in mind:

- **Be comfortable in using active listening skills.** These are the basic skills of counselling and involve the ability to be empathic, non-judgemental and focussed on the perspective of the person with whom you are working and genuine within relationships.
- **Remember that it is not your role to take people's feelings away.** As a course facilitator, you will need to be able to discuss people's emotions and difficulties while allowing them to feel sad or frustrated: people sometimes need to be able to explore such emotions, and the aim of the course is to create a safe place for people with dementia to do this. You, therefore, need to feel able to let people explore and express their emotions without taking them away from this. We will explain more about what we mean by this in the course of the workbook.
- **Find support for yourself.** Running a *Living Well with Dementia* course is hard work. You will need to be supported by colleagues and have regular supervision if you are to be able to reflect on what has happened, build your own confidence as a facilitator and improve your skills. You should also look after yourself to make sure that you

are able to deal with the emotions and problems this type of work often raises.

- **Find support for the course.** Talking to others within your service will also help them understand the support you are providing and know who to refer to you. The *Living Well with Dementia* approach brings a relatively novel and different way of thinking. The focus on working with the person and their family to achieve empowerment and active coping skills is rather different from the traditional way of focussing on the management of dementia symptoms rather than on the person. Consequently, not all health and social care professionals fully understand the idea of working therapeutically with people with dementia rather than just giving advice. You may need to take an evangelical approach to spreading the word!

Selection and recruitment of course participants

As we have mentioned, not everyone who has dementia will benefit from attending a *Living Well with Dementia* course. In order to be able to participate and benefit from being part of a course, participants will need to have:

- **Sufficient cognitive ability to benefit from attending.** Participants need to have sufficient cognitive capacity to consent to be involved in the group and to benefit from the discussions. For this reason, in previous research studies, we have specified that participants have a mild or moderate level of dementia – for instance, scoring above 18 on the MMSE (Mini-Mental State Examination; Folstein, Folstein & McHugh, 1975). However, this is not a hard-and-fast rule. We have found that some people with higher scores, but who found it hard to engage, get less from the course than do people with lower scores, but who clearly want to talk about what has happened in their lives.
- **A diagnosis of dementia.** The course is aimed specifically at people who have been given a diagnosis of dementia – whether this is Alzheimer's disease, vascular or Lewy body dementia. For this reason, people with a diagnosis of Mild Cognitive Impairment (MCI) or people who do not have a diagnosis should not be offered the course. People who have co-morbid diagnoses of dementia and other health conditions (such as Parkinson's disease) can be included if they meet the other criteria that we set out – but do consider how you might be able to meet any significant sensory or physical health needs that they have.

  Generally speaking, people who have received a diagnosis of frontal-temporal dementia (FTD) may struggle to gain much from the group for two reasons: first, they may well struggle to empathise with the perspectives or with others in the group, and second, some of the specific guidance on the course doesn't relate to them. However, we know of some people with this diagnosis, especially the temporal variant of FTD, who both gain from attending the course and contribute fully to the group. So, again, recruitment needs to be made on a case-by-case basis using your own clinical judgement.

- **Awareness that they have been given a diagnosis of dementia.** Potential participants don't have to refer to their diagnosis directly – they may, for instance, talk about "it" or "that thing". They may also be inconsistent in how they talk about it, sometimes completely dismissing it while at other times grudgingly acknowledging that they do have a memory problem. However, what is important is that a potential participant does not completely avoid the subject or show such high levels of distress when others bring it up that it is clear that discussing these themes will be too much for them to tolerate.

- **Capacity to tolerate some distress.** This is a crucial, but difficult to assess, issue. This is because coming to a *Living Well with Dementia* course does mean having to talk about dementia, which can bring up distressing feelings. In essence, deciding whether someone should be part of a course means trying to make a decision about whether they have the psychological and social resources necessary to tolerate the distress that engaging with their diagnosis brings with it. This judgement is separate to the judgements we make about intellectual or cognitive capacity. However, in general, we take a position of assuming that people do have the emotional capacity to benefit from a *Living Well with Dementia* course, just as we would assume that people had the intellectual capacity to give consent, unless there is evidence to the contrary. In making a decision about a person's capacity to talk about their dementia, some of the areas you might want to consider are:

  - **Their social relationships.** For instance, if their family actively opposes talking about dementia, then other options are likely to be more appropriate – for instance, working with them as a couple. Other things to bear in mind are whether there is someone who is able to support the person or who can discuss issues that come up with them and help them to deal with any practical issues that come up, for instance, helping them to get to the course.

  - **The person's own psychological resilience to distress.** You will need to think about whether they have a significant pre-morbid history of functional mental health problems such as psychosis or a major depression, which might indicate that they will find it difficult to tolerate the emotions that the course might arouse. More generally, you need to be able to think about the extent to which someone can tolerate a threat to their self-esteem or identity, including their ability to manage change. Sometimes, people whose sense of self-esteem comes from what they have achieved in life, rather than from whom they are, may be too emotionally fragile to benefit from thinking about the losses involved in dementia.

- **Interest in and willingness to attend a course** and discuss their feelings within a group session. You will need to be open with potential participants that attending the course will involve being with others who have dementia, and therefore they will need to be able to listen to people talking about their experiences.

- **Sufficient communication skills** to enable them to participate in group discussions. This may mean that some people with dysphasia, or who have severe hearing loss (and are not willing or not able to wear a hearing aid) or who have very limited ability to speak in English may not benefit from attending the course. There are no hard-and-fast rules about this: often people who have very obvious communication problems, but who nevertheless are very motivated and willing to engage with their illness, can be important and valuable members of a course. So, again, you will need to think about this on a case-by-case basis.

- **Commitment to attending regular meetings.** Participants don't have to come to every session of the course, but attending the first two or three sessions is especially important, as it is during this time that the group establishes itself and people get to know each other.

- **Composition of the group – age, ethnicity and gender.** Typically, it is best if at least two people on a course share a characteristic. So if there is only one man, or a single female, in a group, this may contribute to the person feeling isolated. This consideration also relates to other visible characteristics such as age and ethnicity: people with young-onset dementia or from a BAME community may have very different concerns from older, white participants, and consequently, you will need to think about the balance of participants attending the course. Sometimes it may be preferable to defer entry onto the course to a later time, when you can ensure that there is a more even balance of participants.

It is very important to meet all the participants yourself to see if the group will be right for them and to gauge whether they will "gel" with the other people on the course. Meet each potential participant with their partner or close family member to talk about the groups. Take enough time to explain the aims, processes and potential benefits as well as disadvantages of taking part in the groups. Give people a good opportunity to ask any questions and ensure they are making an informed choice about whether to take part in the groups. Check whether they have any sensory or other difficulties to help you plan the sessions.

You may need to start with a list of twice as many potential participants as you need in order to end up with a final group of six to eight people.

Practical issues in setting up a course

- **Dynamic administration.** The time that you invest outside the course in making sure that it happens is just as important as what you do within sessions. Every participant needs to know when the groups are on and how they get there, and you will often need to stay engaged with participants and their families before the group starts and during the group itself. If people live on their own, then they may need regular phone calls to remind them about sessions. A common reason why a course struggles is because the administrative work behind the scenes is neglected or ignored. (NB: Just because this is "administration", don't leave this to a junior person in the team!)

- **Transport to the sessions.** Facilitators may need to help participants to organise transport. The location needs to be easily accessible by public transport, including for people who have a physical disability.

- **Finding a suitable room and setting it up.** The room should be large enough for all participants to sit comfortably in a circle, move around a little and have refreshments in the room rather than outside. There should also be good light. The room may need to be accessible for people who have mobility considerations.

- **Awareness of diversity issues.** It is important for facilitators to think of how they can make the course equally appropriate to everyone from their community. You may need to think about the practical arrangements that will need to be made to the course to ensure all people can use it – for instance, whether an interpreter is needed or making yourself aware of particular issues for people from BAME communities. There may be people from different BAME communities who might benefit from a *Living Well with Dementia* course but who don't access local dementia services. You could talk to organisers of any community groups specifically catering to the needs of people from BAME communities and see if they think running a course for people attending their organisation might be possible. If so, then don't be afraid to make changes to how the course is set out – discuss with the organisers what is likely to be useful, what might need to be altered or even left out completely and what might need to be added.

- **Materials and resources.** Think about visual aids such as a flip chart but also plan what you will do for people who have visual and hearing impairments. All of the handouts for the sessions are in the appendix at the back of this workbook, and they will also be available as e-resources to download from www.routledge\9781138542358.

- **Support from others in your service.** A course doesn't exist in a vacuum – you need everyone who you work with to be signed on to the idea of the course and to promote and respect its aims. For instance, your colleagues need to make sure that you are not disturbed or interrupted during a session. Students or visitors should be allowed to observe sessions only after discussion with group members and ensuring they are really comfortable with this. Often, having someone new in the group environment can be destabilising.

- **Co-facilitation.** You will need a co-facilitator with whom you have a good trusting relationship so you can support each other. A lot goes on during a course, and two people can manage all the group processes much more effectively than one. Two leaders can better ensure that the required attention is paid to participants' emotional and psychological well-being, while keeping on track with the planned structure and processes. Having two leaders can also ensure continuality of groups in unforeseen circumstances, such as sickness.

- **Planning.** Take time before each session to discuss which co-facilitator will do what. Will you take turns to lead or will one person lead while the other observes? Also allow time at the end for reflection and learning points. Be open with each other about your differences in style or approach and try to find a way to resolve differences that come up with which you are both comfortable.

- **Note-taking and de-briefing.** Make sure that you and your co-facilitator have enough time at the end of the group to talk about what has happened. So *do not schedule other work for at least an hour after the group finishes*! There will be a need to clear up after the group, but you will also need to write your notes together (both for individual participants and for the course as a whole) and agree if there are issues that need to be thought about the following week. This is likely to involve the practical (making a note of anyone who can't attend, or remembering that one course member didn't say much, perhaps because they couldn't hear) and also the more general (for instance, what issues came up that were difficult or emotive).

- **Supervision.** No matter how experienced or trained you are, you will need to have a space where you can discuss your clinical work and the issues that it brings up for you personally and for your clients. This supervision needs to be a joint activity with both facilitators attending supervision sessions with a supervisor together. Ideally, this needs to be someone who has experience of running groups or similar courses – regardless of whether this is with people with dementia. It should also be someone with whom you are both comfortable. As your work on the course starts long before the first session, your supervision should not only cover the period of the course itself, but also should guide you through the process of assessing potential participants and the pre-planning necessary for the course to run smoothly. Ideally, supervision should occur at monthly, if not weekly, intervals.

Involving members of the family

Working with the family is crucial to the success of the course but can create a significant dilemma: without family support, the impact of the course group is significantly undermined, but at the same time, the course is structured so that the majority of the sessions involves only people who are living with a diagnosis of dementia. Sometimes carers can feel somewhat left out of the course, but there are two reasons why we believe it is important to focus the sessions solely on the person with dementia:

- First, our experience has been that when the person with dementia attends a session with their partner or a member of their family, they often look to that person to speak for them, and thus we do not hear their own voice.

• Second, many participants have strong feelings around their relationships that they need to be free to explore. Almost always, however, the person who is living with dementia has very mixed feelings – grateful for the support and love they are shown, yet also being aware of another side to their feelings. Typically, they may feel guilty about the increased burden that now falls on their partner, or they may simply not want to worry their family by acknowledging just how much in their life has changed. Very occasionally, they may also feel annoyed or frustrated by aspects of their relationships.

It is important, then, to provide a safe enough space for people who are living with dementia to explore their emotions and to listen to other members of the course do the same. At the same time, we want to make sure that the families are as involved in the course as possible, and we can do this by:

• **Using the handouts.** The course handouts are an essential way of communicating with partners and members of the family. It is, therefore, vital that you encourage families and partners to discuss the issues on the handout with course participants and to work together on the material completing the exercises as appropriate.

• **The preliminary meeting.** During this meeting, the person with dementia is joined by their partner or another member of their family or a friend. This is a crucial session, as it is during this meeting that you will be able to outline what is involved in coming to the groups and introduce the ethos of the course – that although coming together to discuss experiences is often difficult, it helps people to accept and to adjust to change. Consequently, you can explain that you will have an expectation that families or couples find time to discuss the material in the handouts after each session, and that if they have any concerns or queries, then they should get in touch with you. During the preliminary meeting, you may also need to deal with any anxieties family members might have about the person with dementia attending the course and explaining how they can provide support.

• **The post-course group meeting.** During this meeting, you should encourage partners to continue to provide support with the material covered in the course and give you their feedback about any changes they have noticed. It also provides a chance for you to briefly (and without breaking confidentiality) discuss what have been the main issues and to present the perspectives of the course attendees.

• **Parallel family meetings.** Occasionally, if resources allow, it may be possible for a service to run a parallel session for family members that takes place while the main course is running. However, as we know that for most NHS services, resources are stretched, we do not specify that this has to occur. If there are sufficient resources to allow, then these discussions should ideally be led by a health care professional and allow a balance of discussing the carers' own needs and addressing the material covered within the main course. If resources are not sufficient to allow this, then it may be possible to encourage carers who are bringing and collecting participants to meet and provide a mutual self-help group, for instance, in a local café.

Course leadership skills

Talking about dementia and the problems it causes is important because people can gain insight into their situation. On the course, participants can help each other to accept the situation and learn ways to cope with some of the changes. However, discussing difficult issues before participants are ready to do so can be distressing and mean that the course feels unsafe.

For the first couple of sessions, then, it may be better to talk to the group in general terms about "memory problems" rather than use the term "dementia". At the same time, if somebody on the course uses the terms "Alzheimer's disease" or "dementia", then you need to be ready to talk directly about the illness. This is important, because coming into the course can also help people to overcome some of their fears about dementia. As Robert, a participant in an early version of the course who had initially been reluctant to talk about his dementia, said (Watkins et al., 2006):

> *I find I've got a great deal of moral uplift by coming here. Meeting you, listening to the way you do it. And I don't see the problem now, it frightened me, the problem of declining memory, until I came here, and now I'm not frightened. . . . Because I thought, well, I'm going mad, I'm going crazy. What am I going to be like in another five years? But now I realize that everybody is getting this problem.*

As the course progresses, so you can start to slowly explore how memory loss and other cognitive problems affect people and how it makes them feel. The emphasis is on helping the group to share their experiences together, to learn that they are not alone and to help course participants to gain confidence in talking about this difficult subject together.

You can help people realise that they share similar problems by pointing out where participants are describing similar experiences. At the same time, try not to leave out people whose experiences are different. For instance, some people may struggle to get words out due to dysphasia, while others may be different because of age, gender or race. Think very carefully if you have people with young-onset dementia who may still be working or trying to work and have relatively young families. If there isn't someone else on the course who is like them, then they are likely to feel isolated. Make sure that differences between participants are remembered and discussed openly within the course in as supportive and empathic a way as possible.

Discussing the experiences of memory problems can be stressful. Be gentle and do not push people to talk if they are reluctant. Be aware of anyone on the course who has a problem talking about dementia. If someone is quiet and doesn't speak, then remember to check out how they are feeling.

Key points

- Be positive – help participants to view their difficulties realistically but explore ways of reducing disability, encouraging people not to give up and to build on past successes.
- Provide guidance only when necessary – try to remember this simple phrase: *ASK: DON'T TELL* (see our discussion of the research evidence around this in Chapter 1). All too often course inexperienced facilitators make the mistake of leaping ahead and telling participants what they might be thinking.
- Encourage participants to communicate with each other and to share similar feelings and experiences – try asking *"Mr X was saying. . . . What do other people think?"*
- Be the "memory" for the group – remember what people have said and come back to it, when you can.
- Ask for more information – try using a prompt such as *"that was interesting – tell me more"*.
- Allow participants to express and experience strong emotions – even negative ones, such as anger and shame.
- Support altruism – encourage participants to help each other out, but make sure that they don't talk on behalf of each other.
- Encourage talking in first person (*"I feel . . ."*) rather than with distance (for instance, *"One feels . . ."* or *"Everyone feels . . ."*).
- Be aware that there may be times when you need to move ahead to another section of the course and use some of the material at an earlier stage. For instance, sometimes course participants can become impatient and want to start talking about dementia at an earlier stage. If this happens, then don't feel that you have to stick rigorously to the order of the chapters as we have set them out – instead, if you feel comfortable doing so and feel that the group is ready to move on, then do vary the order in which you cover these topics.

Course development

Throughout the course, pay attention to the stage of the course and adapt your facilitation style accordingly.

- In the beginning sessions, participants are getting to know each other and how the course will operate. Facilitators need to provide a lot of structure in this phase to encourage cohesion and to make people feel safe.

- During the middle sessions, course participants are likely to be able to work more actively on the problems and issues that concern them. This phase often feels like the most productive stage of the course, as participants talk more openly about their experiences. Facilitators need to take more of a back seat, just promoting and encouraging people to engage with the material.

- As the course nears its end, facilitators should prepare participants and help them think about future support and options for keeping in touch with others. At the end of the group, make sure to find some way of marking the contribution that each member has made. Recognise the successes of the group, while also allowing the group to be disappointed that it is ending.

Including a maintenance or follow-up session

The *Living Well with Dementia* course does not specifically suggest that facilitators create a follow-up session, because we understand that resources are often stretched. However, there are potential benefits in doing so – for instance, it helps participants to maintain any progress and lessens the sense of feeling abandoned that some may experience. If you do decide to organise a maintenance session, then organising this for six to ten weeks after the end of the course is often the best timing. Let participants and their partners know about the arrangements for such a meeting in the final session.

If you do go ahead with a maintenance session, then it is likely that the content of the session will be relatively minimal: it will offer participants a chance to catch up with each other and with you, while it gives you a chance to find out if any of the commitments or ideas from the course have been followed through on.

Using the workbook

In using the workbook, there are a few important points to bear in mind.

Training

In writing the workbook, we have tried to ensure that all of the most important ingredients in leading a *Living Well with Dementia* course have been addressed. If the suggestions that we make are followed, then in most circumstances, the workbook can, therefore, be used as a stand-alone guide. However, where possible, we would recommend that potential course facilitators seek out appropriate training. This may take different forms: first, many health care professions see running a support group or educational course as a core element of their professional training – and this is why we anticipate that many course facilitators will have their own background knowledge and skills in this area to draw on. Second, it is possible to attend many continuing professional development courses that will help to build up skills in this area, even if they don't specifically relate to working with people with dementia. Finally, at the time of writing, a two-day training package specifically designed to develop the skills needed by *Living Well with Dementia* course facilitators is run twice a year at the University of the West of England – more details can be found at www1.uwe.ac.uk/study/professionaldevelopment.aspx.

Other resources

In the workbook, we refer on a number of occasions to resources which (at the time of our writing this manual) can be found online. We realise that these materials are all UK focussed and we apologise if, at times, referring to UK law or policies (for instance, those around the blue badge parking scheme) are not relevant to readers outside the UK. One other resource, which we don't specifically refer to in the workbook, may also be worth pursuing – this is a set of short films made for a precursor of the course called *Memory Matters*. These films were created by Ann Marshall and her colleagues at Southern Health, and can be found at www. southernhealth.nhs.uk/services/mental-health/older/memory-matters/memory-matters-films/.

Different voices

This workbook is intended to be read by course facilitators. At times, however, we suggest a form of words that could be used by facilitators to address course participants – and when we do that, we use italics to distinguish the voice of the authors addressing facilitators and one possible voice that facilitators may choose to use to address course participants. In doing this, we would like to emphasise that this is simply our suggestion for how you might want to frame the activity to participants. We are aware that a risk in writing the manual in this way is that facilitators may feel constrained to read out precisely what we have written, as if it were a script for a play. This is *not* what we want you to do! We simply hope that it gives you an idea of the sort of things you could say. The most important thing is that you, as a course facilitator, find your own words to address these issues.

We want to share one final thought with you. We hope you find this workbook helpful to you in running a *Living Well with Dementia* course. They are hard work – it can be mentally and emotionally exhausting to run a course. There are many challenges, from putting the course together, to balancing keeping the course running while also responding to issues that come up. However, our experience is that working in this way can also be enormously rewarding. We would like to finish with some quotations from course facilitators in our pilot study which summarise what we often hear.

That, you know, you've worked with these people and they've got something out of it, some more than others, but they've all got something, they've taken something away. And you just feel as if you've really achieved something. So I think it's the reward is huge.

You know, you're often looking for little things, you're not, you know with dementia you're not looking for huge great leaps and changes and you often have to put a lot of work in to get something back from people but when you see that I think that really makes you feel like you've done something.

Oh I enjoyed meeting the people, their personalities and, you know, they'd often talk about their history, which we encouraged, about their life experiences and what they did for jobs and very diverse roles from air hostesses and . . . [laughing] amazing lives. . . . It's just a joy to get to know them and a privilege really.

3 Preliminary meeting for participants and partners

Session summary

Aim. The purpose of this session is to introduce the ethos of the intervention and to outline what is involved in coming to the groups. The session should both provide reassurance and also make plain to participants what will be involved in coming to the course.

Context. The primary purpose of the *Living Well with Dementia* course is that bringing people who are living with dementia (and their families) together to discuss their experiences helps people to adjust to their problems. It is also important to deal with any anxieties that participants or their friend or family member might have about attending the groups.

Process. It is important to welcome and introduce participants and their partners so they feel that you are interested in their experiences. Facilitators will need to agree roles before the session starts.

Content. Initially, we will focus on introductions and getting to know each other, then discuss the practicalities of attending and group rules before moving on to introduce the *Living Well with Dementia* course. The key messages about the course that need to be communicated are that (i) attendance at each week is important, and (ii) that the work between sessions (based around reading and discussing the handouts together) is a vital part of the course.

Activity 1: welcome and ice-breaker exercise

Pre-meeting preparation

Arrive in time to prepare the room properly with the correct number and same type of chairs for the expected number of participants. Arrange chairs so that people can see the flip charts. Provide tea and coffee that people can drink before the group starts, and make sure the group starts promptly. As it is the first week, it may be welcoming to make the tea and coffee for people and hand it to them, but if people want to help themselves or others to tea and coffee, that is fine. At the same time, you will

Table 3.1 Session plan for the preliminary meeting with participants and partners

Objective	Activity	Duration	Resources	Expected outcome
To introduce the course and its aims.	Welcome and ice-breaker	30 min	Tea and coffee, name badges, marker and flip chart	Participants and partners should feel more comfortable and relaxed after getting to know others.
To help participants learn about the ethos of the course.	What does "living well with dementia" mean?	15 min		Participants will understand more about the course.
To get participants and their families to "buy into" the concept of the course and get them to talk about it together.	Explain what participants can get out of coming on the course	30 min	Handouts, folders, flip chart and marker	Participants should understand the purpose of the course and how this can help them.
To outline the importance of attending and discussing the sessions at home. Explore whether relatives and friends can meet.	Finish up the session	15 min		Participants and relatives and friends understand the importance of working together at home using the handouts and making practical arrangements.

need to keep an eye on how the participants with dementia pour any hot water and be ready to step in if there are unnecessary risks. If you are using name badges, then make sure they are large enough for people to read.

Introduction

Make sure that you know the names of everyone who is going to be attending and any health and safety housekeeping issues that need to be flagged. After welcoming everyone, move fairly quickly into the first activity.

Ice-breaker: how did people get here?

✓ Ask each pair to talk to the couple next to them (or people that they do not yet know) about their journey to the group.
✓ Suggest that the pairs agree who will go first, and that each couple has a pen and paper to make a note of what they have been told if they

wish. This should take a few minutes for each couple, before you ask them to switch over.

✓ Then ask each pair to introduce their neighbours to the larger group. Try to get the person with dementia to do the feeding back, but be aware that some may find this difficult and may need prompting and support.

Activity 2: what does "living well with dementia" mean?

Explain to the group that in this course, we will focus on "living well" with dementia. What we mean by this is that we want to help people living with dementia and their family to live as fulfilling a life as they can despite the difficulties and challenges that they face because of the illness.

Talking with other people who are going through similar experiences is important because that is the way in which we learn that we're not alone. But this is also difficult – sometimes it's only natural to want to forget about difficult things.

In the groups we will talk at times about "living well" as we know that there is no cure for dementia. However, dementia not only affects skills like someone's memory, but also impacts on them in other ways. Sometimes people lose confidence in themselves, or they change how the live their life. For instance, people may stop going shopping because they find it difficult to remember what they need to buy or because they are worried they will be confused when it comes to paying. Often, people don't know whether to tell other people about their dementia, or what to say. Coming to the group won't help you to have a better memory, but we hope that by discussing the illness with other people, so you will be able to find ways to be more confident and that this will improve your quality of life – and help you to live better.

We believe the best way to do this is to:

✓ *Adjust to what has changed and learn how to live with it*
✓ *Hold on to hope and have a sense of meaning and purpose*
✓ *Make decisions about how things are now and how you would like them to be in the future*
✓ *Find a way around problems that come up*
✓ *Feel part of life rather than feeling shut out of it*

During the course of the groups, we will:

✓ *Encourage you to share your experiences*
✓ *Help you to feel more confident in thinking and talking about your problems*
✓ *Talk about how to live as well as possible even with these problems – for instance, to think about making decisions about your lives*

In order to achieve these aims, we need families to play their part in supporting the group by:

✓ *Looking through the handouts with the participant and talking them over with participants*
✓ *Doing some of the exercises (for instance, relaxation and memory prompts) together*

We would like to encourage both the participants on the course and their partners to read through the handouts at home. Talk to your partners about the handouts and try the exercises. These will remind you about the most important aspects of the course and help you to use the ideas that we have discussed at home. Discussing the handouts at home together is an important part of the course.

Activity 3: what can you get out of coming here?

The purpose of this exercise is for participants and their partners to talk to each other about what they hope to get out of the participant coming to the course. This will also help people start to get to know each other.

At the start of this activity, distribute the folders and the handouts for this session to each couple. Briefly talk through the main points that it covers which you have not already addressed and go over the structure of the course and what future sessions will involve, although not in great detail at this point.

While one facilitator leads feedback from participants, the other can write the notes up on a flip chart. Put positive thoughts on the left hand side, concerns on the right.

Ask each pair to talk to the couple next to them about their thoughts on:

✓ What they hope to get out of coming on the course
✓ Any concerns they may have about coming here

After about five minutes, ask people to share their ideas with the group. Write people's feedback up on a flip chart. Respond to the concerns and reinforce realistic expectations.

As this is the first session and people are likely to be very anxious, go slowly and carefully. However, in writing the feedback, take any opportunities that arise to gently tease out from couples any aspects of living well with dementia that you may need to return to later on, such as:

✓ Whether the person with dementia has lost confidence
✓ Whether their behaviour has changed – for instance, not going out as much
✓ Any ideas or goals about how they would like to change life

Finish up the session

To conclude the session, you need to do two key things.

First, you need to describe how your administrative arrangements will work. Emphasise that people should commit to the groups every week – and tell people the arrangements for contacting you if they can't attend (make sure that you add your contact details to the handout for this session). You also need to let participants and partners know how they can contact you if they have any concerns about issues or discussions that have happened during the course. It is much better that people who do have concerns contact you to discuss them, rather than stay quiet. You should also reassure participants that it may take a few weeks for them to feel comfortable about coming, but that most people who attend the *Living Well with Dementia* course feel that they benefit and are glad that they came.

The second thing that you need to do is to discuss whether it is possible for partners to meet each other while the *Living Well with Dementia* sessions are going on. If it is not possible for your team to run a parallel carers' course, then perhaps partners and family could, for example, meet up every week in a local café, or find some other way to support each other.

4 Session 1: is there anything wrong with me?

Aim. The key activity for today is for people to feel that the course is a safe place to share the problems and frustrations they experience and to bond with the other course members by acknowledging similar experiences or concerns.

Context. This is the first of eight sessions that participants will be attending alone, without their partners. Talking about dementia and the problems it causes is important because people can gain insight into their situation. They can learn to accept the situation and learn ways to help them cope with some of the changes.

Process. Discussing difficult issues before the group is ready to do so can be distressing and mean that the group feels unsafe. For the first couple of sessions, then, it may be better to talk to the group in general terms about "memory problems" rather than to use the term "dementia". At the same time, if somebody on the course uses the terms "Alzheimer's disease" or "dementia", then you need to be ready to talk directly about this with the group and to adapt your approach.

Content. After the initial welcome and ice-breaker activity, briefly remind people about the course rules that you set up in the first meeting before setting out the reasons why people are here. The main activity in this session is aimed at slowly exploring how memory loss and other cognitive problems affect participants. The emphasis is on helping the group to share their experiences together, to learn that they are not alone and to help participants to gain confidence in talking about this difficult subject. As some participants are likely to be nervous about being on the course, reassure them that feeling anxious is normal and that the aim of the course is to help them to feel better and more confident.

Activity 1: welcome and ice-breaker exercise

Make sure that you welcome participants by name to the course.

An ice-breaking activity is an important part of the session to help participants relax and feel more comfortable talking to other people in

Table 4.1 Session plan for week one – is there anything wrong with me?

Objective	Activity	Duration	Resources	Expected outcome
To set out the principles of the course, to help participants relax and get to know others.	Ice-breaker Course rules	10 min 10 min	Participants' ideas, this handbook, flip chart and marker	This exercise helps participants know the course better, but mainly helps you engage everyone in making this "their" course.
To address any concerns about today's session.	Introduction, reminder of previous week's activity and identifying any worries	10 min	Last week's flip charts, new flip chart and marker	This helps participants to remember the aims of the course and facilitators to identify expectations and worries.
To explore participants' experiences of living with dementia.	Is there anything wrong with me?	60 min	This handbook, flip chart and marker	Participants start talking about dementia and the problems they have because of it, as well as things they still do well.

the group. Even though participants will have met in the previous session, an ice-breaker can still free people up to talk to each other and prepare them for the session.

Ice-breaker: hopes and fears

After the preliminary meeting where the course was introduced, people might have some fears and expectations about attending that might have been forgotten or not discussed before. Provide the group with paper and pens (helping any people who struggle with writing) and split the group into pairs or threes. Then ask them to:

- Introduce themselves.
- Discuss one thing that they were nervous or concerned about or looking forward to in coming today to a course called *Living Well with Dementia*.
- Allow each pair to talk for about five minutes – try to listen in to check how things are going and if there are problems. Then encourage each pair to feedback. Use the flip chart and write people's concerns on the left and things they were looking forward to on the right.

Tip. One reason why participants may be nervous about being on the course is that their dementia makes it harder to remember names or why they are in the meeting and so on. You might want to explore this with the group.

Introduction

Today we will start talking about your experiences with memory problems or dementia and how you cope with any problems that come up. We also want to think about the things you still do well.

First of all, it's normal to be apprehensive and worried about coming to groups, especially if the focus is a sensitive topic such as memory loss or dementia. It is also normal that people feel worried about starting any new thing. However, we want the groups to be friendly and we hope that you will be able to relax and feel welcome.

Activity 2: set up your own group rules

Now it's time to agree about how we will behave during the course. We want to make sure that everyone feels welcome, safe and free to say ideas without judgement. What rules would you suggest that we have and follow during the sessions?

Here are some suggestions:

✓ *Confidentiality – what is said in the group stays in the group*
✓ *Attendance – it is important to come to all sessions and let someone know if cannot make it*
✓ *Listening and talking – one person to speak at a time*
✓ *Balance listening and talking – everyone gets a turn*
✓ *Everyone's opinion is important – no judging of people or their opinions*
✓ *Don't speak for other people – they may have different experiences*
✓ *Equal opportunity for everyone to speak*

Every course needs a set of rules to be run by. Course rules can help participants understand the expectations about their behaviour while they are in the group. It is good practice when participants make and agree upon the rules with the leader's assistance. It supports group dynamics and helps people to feel more in control, which is what we want to achieve. You can think about a way of making the rules visible in the group – for instance, participants could bring a copy of these each week in their folder, or you could have the rules visible in the room each week.

Handout

Distribute today's handouts and suggest that people can write down some ideas from the session. Remind participants that the handouts are important and that reading through them at home with partners will help them to get the most out of the course.

Activity 3: is there anything wrong with me?

The main activity for today is to get people to discuss the problems and frustrations they have as a result of their dementia. The title of today's session is "Is there anything wrong with me?". This is because one way that many people have of coping with dementia is to ignore or to down-play their problems. People say things like "I can still do everything I used to do" or "I do have a poor memory, but no more so than anyone else who is my age". The aim of today is not to challenge these ideas directly. Instead, we want the group to share their views together.

You should have about 30 minutes for this activity. Start by reminding people of the importance of sharing their experience and then encourage the group to talk about their experience with dementia. The activity is to ask people to list what they do well and then what memory and other problems they have.

Sharing our experiences and problems we go through is very important. Talking about problems that we have can not only help us understand our own experience better but also cope with the illness and find ways to live with it. Now we will start talking about how the memory problems of dementia affect your life and the things you do well.

Ask the group to list:

✓ The things that haven't changed and that people still enjoy or are good at
✓ The memory and other problems people may have experienced

You may find it works best to ask people first to discuss the issues in pairs for about 10–15 minutes. You can join each pair for a minute to support them and see how they are doing. If people have difficulties sharing experiences or if they become distressed, provide emotional support. Alternatively, it might work best staying with the whole group for this discussion.

Then, in the whole group, ask for examples. You will first simply write up a list of what they tell you on a flip chart (for instance, write up problems on the left, and things that haven't changed and that people still enjoy or are good at on the right). This will help people realise there are both positive and negative aspects.

As you do this, help participants to realise that they share similar problems by pointing out where participants are describing similar experiences. These could include feeling confused or muddled, forgetting names, phone numbers, where they live or how to get home; and difficulties in doing everyday tasks, such as handling money.

At the same time, try not to leave out people whose experiences are different. For instance, some people may struggle to get words out due to dysphasia, while others may be different because of age, gender or culture. Make sure that these differences are remembered and acknowledged within the group in as supportive and empathic a way as possible.

Many thanks for coming to today's session. We have looked at the sorts of problems that memory difficulties/dementia creates for people – it sounds as if some of these difficulties are shared by everyone here – and some of them are relevant only for one or two people.

What is important is how these problems make you feel – not being able to remember names, for instance, may make you feel more nervous when you come to meetings like this, for instance. Often, when people are anxious, they do less – they may end up avoiding going shopping or meeting friends. But when that happens, they lose more confidence, and become more fed up. This can end up being a vicious circle.

This is what we will come back to in later sessions.

Are there any questions?

Finish up the session

To finish up the session, return to the fears and expectations people described in the beginning. Look again at the flip chart and encourage the group to discuss their views about the session. Find out whether all of these fears are still relevant, or whether they are held as strongly.

Finally, thank participants for their contribution to the group and for sharing their thoughts and feelings. Remind them the date and time of the next session, check that everyone can attend and ask if there any questions.

5 Session 2: memory aids and strategies

Session summary

Aim. In the first session, the group talked about the problems that arise as a result of dementia as well as the things they still do well. Today, we will build on this by talking about how memory works and what participants can do that will help them to remember important things. We will take opportunities to gently make the link between the impact of memory loss (and other problems associated with dementia) and how this makes people feel. The session involves both recognising and empathising with the difficulties people have as a result of their illness and beginning to suggest strategies that could help people live everyday lives.

Context. This session is part of the group continuing to form – it is still relatively early in the process of the group coming together. The focus of the session is, therefore, on a task (identifying memory strategies) but also includes exercises to build interactions between participants and to help participants to address a central issue in their lives.

Process. While the focus is specifically on memory loss, it is possible that not all participants, depending on their diagnosis, will experience this as their main symptom. It is, therefore, important to be aware of the diagnosis of all participants and to make sure that the discussion is still relevant to them. Any discussion of strategies also needs to build on what people are already doing – for instance, whether they use diaries, calendars, tablets, phones or other aids.

Content. After telling the group about housekeeping and reminding them about the course rules, start with a short ice-breaker activity. Then hold a short interactive group discussion about what had been discussed in the previous session and give people the handouts to use during today's session and write in any notes or ideas from the activities about memory loss and aids. When finishing up, remember to return to the worries and expectations that you discussed in the beginning. Explore how people feel and whether any worries were cleared up.

Table 5.1 Session plan for week two – memory aids and strategies

Objective	Activity	Duration	Resources	Expected outcome
To help participants relax in the session.	Ice-breaker: the name game	15 min	This handbook, a hat or bag, sticky labels, pens	Participants relax, know other participants on the course and feel comfortable enough to share their experiences.
To remind participants about last week's activity and prepare for today.	Reminder: problems and strengths	15 min	Last week's flip chart, marker	Participants remember what they talked about last week and recall the problems they experience due to their illness and what they still do well.
To talk about memory and explore the ways we can help it. To suggest some memory aids to try out.	How your memory works? How to make things "stick" – memory aids and strategies?	15 min 20 min	This handbook, handouts	Participants know more about how their memory works and what to expect. Help them recognise the need for extra effort to remember things.
To look at emotions relating to memory.	What makes it hard to think about memory problems? Marjory (optional activity)	25 min	This handbook, handouts, flip chart and marker	Participants open up a little and explore the opportunity to talk about their problems, including feeling confused, frightened or sad.

Activity 1: the name game

If you have been using name badges, then ask participants to put these in a hat or a bag. If you haven't used name badges, then write these out on sticky labels. Then let each person pick one out and read out the name. Ask them to find the person it belongs to and give them the name badge. If participants are uncertain, then reassure them that this is normal – it is a memory group after all!

The first thing we are going to do today is to take off all of your name badges and to place them in this bag. We are then going to go round and everyone in turn will take a name out of the bag and try and find out who it belongs to!

This exercise acts as an ice-breaker and will hopefully increase participants' confidence in the group. However, it is also likely to be one in which people make mistakes – this may allow you the opportunity to notice the mistake and to have a discussion about it if people feel comfortable – for instance, to ask people if they sometimes worry about making these sorts of mistakes. If so, would they avoid situations where they might make a mistake, or do they push on regardless?

Activity 2: introduction

Today we will talk about your memory and how it works. We will explore the problems you experience and the things that you can remember better. We will talk about how memory works and look into the different ways for you to remember important things.

Before we do that however, we need to quickly recap what we spoke about last week (at this point, you might want to bring out the flip chart from week one). *The main points that we discussed were:*

- ✓ *The main problems people here commonly come up against*
- ✓ *The things you do well*

Check whether participants discussed the session and handouts with their partners.

Activity 3: how your memory works

Having explored the problems people have in remembering things, we will now talk about how memory works. Then we will look into what we can do to make it work better (at this point, you might want to distribute the handouts).

One way to think about memory is to distinguish between our immediate and long-term memories. Our short-term memory holds the information that we see or hear for a few seconds. Long-term memory storage holds it for days, months or even years.

As we get older, and particularly if we have problems with our memory, it often becomes harder to move information into long-term storage. The information that was already in long-term storage often tends to stay there, but we have to make more effort to make sure we move new information out from our short-term memory and into the long-term memory.

Dementia almost always makes it harder to move new information into long-term storage, so you may not remember things as well as you used to. Today and in the first session we talked about some problems you have been experiencing.

The process of remembering is a bit like the task of a good secretary or manager. When you see or hear information you would like to memorise, you need to try and move it into the filing cabinet. But all too often it ends up not being neatly filed and is lost or thrown away so that you can't find it when you need it. Putting new information into your long-term memory so that it sticks there is a bit like putting information into a file in a filing cabinet.

Does this ring any bells with you?

Remember, stress and anxiety make things worse. To help you cope with such feelings, we will talk about it in the next few sessions.

Draw a storage cabinet on the flip chart. It doesn't have to be well drawn, but needs to get the point across that new information can be stored away in a filing cabinet and remembered. If it misses the filing cabinet, it ends up on the floor and is forgotten.

How to make things "stick" – using memory strategies

Ask people to talk about what they have tried doing to help them remember important things. Write people's ideas up on a flip chart. This might include "external" aids – things like diaries, calendars and notebooks – as well as "internal" strategies such as repeating things to oneself, going over them or making up a rhyme or pneumonic device (for instance, "Richard Of York Gave Battle In Vain"). (NB: Many people in the course will need support if they are to consistently use these strategies. While this may not be possible for all the course participants, realising that there are ways to improve memory can act as a source of hope even if in reality people don't use the strategies to maximum effect.)

In order to remember new information, it helps if we do something with it in our mind rather than just hearing or seeing it. For instance:

✓ *Organise the information in some way in your mind. For example, write it down. Even if you lose the paper, just the act of having written it down means that you will still have more chance of making it stick in your memory.*

✓ *Make a link between the new information and something familiar you already know. For example, if you meet someone called Peter, you might make the link "Peter Pan" if he looks young.*

✓ *A letter of the alphabet can be a cue – so "P" for "Pea" if Peter has a round face. Once you have the first letter of a name, it acts as a trigger to help you remember it.*

✓ *Repeat it to yourself – but gradually making the gaps between the repetitions longer and longer.*

Remembering it right the first time around will help to reduce mistakes later on, so don't guess, as errors will stick.

Ask the group which of these strategies they have used themselves (following on from earlier discussion) or would like to start using in the future, such as diaries or notebooks, and to write them down (with help if needed on the handout).

OPTIONAL ACTIVITY: MARJORY

Some people in the group may be reluctant to use aids either because they think that having help means that they are giving in or because they don't want to acknowledge they have a problem with their memory. Depending on how well the group has bonded so far, this may be an opportunity to discuss why someone might not want to recognise that they have a poor memory.

Participants may feel able to share their experiences, but if you feel it would be helpful, then you can describe a fictional character ("Marjory") who has some of these qualities: by presenting the discussion as if it were about another person, this may be an indirect way of helping them to think about their own uncertainties. Make sure that

(Continued)

in talking about "Marjory" you let the group know that you're not talking about anyone who is actually a participant (so change the name "Marjory" if there is someone in the group with that name).

I now want to talk about someone who finds it hard to think that she has any problems – let's call her "Marjory", although we could as easily say "Derek" or any other name. Marjory often tells people who she meets that she is getting on really well and that her memory is as sharp now as it's ever been. The only problem is that she sometimes says this three or four times in just 10 minutes and never seems to remember that she has already said it!

- ✓ *Why do you think Marjory says her memory is fine, when she forgets things so easily?*
- ✓ *What do you think might make it hard for Marjory to say that there is something wrong with her memory?*
- ✓ *What might she be feeling?*

Ask people to say what makes it hard for Marjory to talk about her memory problems. Possible responses the group may suggest include:

- ✓ She doesn't think she has changed – this is normal memory loss for someone her age
- ✓ She has good days and bad days
- ✓ She likes to forget about it
- ✓ Her long-term memory is fine, it's just the short-term that is the problem
- ✓ Everyone else is more worried than Marjory, who is just trying to get on with her life
- ✓ She knows she has a problem but doesn't like to think about it because she's worried what others might say about her or she doesn't want to upset them
- ✓ She wants to fight it and doesn't want to give in

Tip. You might want to suggest to the group that Marjory may have mixed feelings – or be in "two minds" about her memory loss. Ask if anyone knows someone like Marjory, and how they would feel about her and what they might want to say to her.

6 Session 3: worry, stress and memory

Session summary

Aim. This session is closely related to the previous session, in which we talked about memory problems and ways of coping. You may already have started to talk about how some participants might prefer (like Marjory) not to talk about their memory problems – for instance, because it might make them feel stressed. This session should, therefore, be seen as following on from the previous week. The aim is to help participants to talk about how their dementia impacts on them, and in particular how it can make people feel stressed and what they can do about it. You can spend some of the first minutes recapping with the group about last week and possibly make links with what was said about people's worries about dementia and how feelings can often lead on to avoidance and a loss of confidence.

Context. In this session, participants will identify how anxiety and stress can arise – for instance, how worry about dementia can lead to avoidance, which, in turn, leads to loss of self-confidence. This is a vicious cycle because anxiety and stress also have a negative effect on memory, which causes more worry, more avoidance and a greater loss of self-confidence – all of which makes it harder to concentrate and to remember. In this session, we will also use a relaxation exercise with the group and look at some thinking strategies that people can use to help them cope with unpleasant and harmful feelings and thoughts.

Process and Content. To start the session, distribute the handouts for this session to everyone and explain that we will be working with them today. Then briefly mention the aims of the session and give a reminder, if you feel it is necessary, of any housekeeping issues and the course rules. You should remind the group that the overall aim is to help them live well with dementia and that using today's main activities and a relaxation exercise will help this process. To finish up, highlight the key points of the session and remind participants to use the handouts at home, discuss it with their partners and to try the exercise at home.

Table 6.1 Session plan for week three – worry, stress and memory

Objective	Activity	Duration	Resources	Expected outcome
To explore how dementia can lead to worry and stress.	Reminder of last session	10 min	Last week's flip chart and marker	Participants are ready to talk about stress.
To talk about how stress affects memory.	Stress and memory	20 min	Flip chart and marker	Participants understand the connection between stress and memory.
To identify more helpful ways of thinking and identify ways to cope with stress.	Discussion	30 min	Flip chart and marker	Participants will be aware of the different ways that they can cope with stress and negative thoughts.
To introduce relaxation exercises and look at how these can be used at home.	Relaxation exercise	30 min	Recording or text of relaxation exercise	Participants have experienced a relaxation exercise and have been given information about resources if they wish to practice relaxation at home.

Activity 1: introduction and review of last week

Today we will continue talking about various problems and feelings that can be related to having dementia. In particular, we will focus on how they can cause worry and stress and how this can affect memory. We will then discuss ways to cope with stress and worries.

As a reminder of last week's activity, put up the flip chart from last week and discuss with the group whether they have been using any of the memory aids and whether they have been helpful.

Activity 2: stress and memory

Usually, a bit of stress is good for us. It makes us energised and focussed. But too much stress is bad and can be harmful. Our bodies respond to too much stress as if we are in danger or under threat. For example:

✓ *Our muscles become tense*
✓ *Our breathing rate increases*
✓ *Our heart beats faster*
✓ *When this happens, it is hard to concentrate, to think clearly and to remember things*

Stress and how we react to it can be like a vicious circle (draw Figure 6.1 on a flip chart).

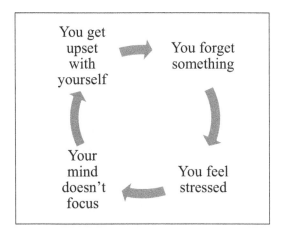

Figure 6.1 The vicious circle of stress and dementia (week three)

As we have discussed before, in order to remember something, we need to concentrate when we hear or read the information. The information is then normally stored in our memory, much like a letter is stored in the correct folder in a filing cabinet, or a library book is placed correctly on a bookcase. However, if we are under a lot of stress, then it is easier to make a mistake in how we put the information into our memory. This means that when we want to remember the information, we can't find it. It's like putting the letter into the wrong folder, or the library book onto the wrong shelf – we're probably not be going to find it when we need it. So learning to cope with stress and anxious feelings may help our memory and help us to feel better.

Activity 3: what do people find stressful and how do they cope?

Now we know that stress not only makes us feel worse but also makes it harder for us to remember things. There are a number of things we can do to cope with stress or worry, some of which are likely to be of more help than others. But before we even cope with stress, we need to first notice that we feel anxious or worried. Once we have done this, then it's useful to identify what we are stressed about. Let's now talk a little about what makes us feel worried, what we do when stressed and how we can cope.

What do you find stressful and worrying?

Write the responses up on a flip chart so people can see and follow the discussion easily. Draw a line down the middle of the flip chart. On the left-hand side of the page, have a column headed "What Makes Me Worried", and on the right-hand side, have a column headed "What I Do to Feel Better". Connect the two with an arrow as we have done in Table 6.2.

Tip. Encourage people to say how the responses of other participants in the group relate to them, so that everyone has a chance to talk.

Table 6.2 Coping with worries about dementia

What makes me worried		What I do to feel better
Not remembering people's names	➤	Bluff it out
Forgetting where I put things	➤	Blame others, become angry
Forgetting what has been said	➤	Not take part
Forgetting what I want to say	➤	Stay quiet
Not being understood	➤	Feel upset
Not doing what I used to do	➤	Withdraw into myself

What to do if you can't remember things

Discuss positive coping strategies and list these on the flip chart. This might include statements such as:

- ✓ If you find yourself worrying about something you have forgotten, then tell yourself it doesn't matter and it will probably come back later. Getting worked up will just make it worse.
- ✓ Try and distract yourself as a way of relaxing. For example:
  - ○ Listen to music
  - ○ Look at things around you and try to focus on what is happening
  - ○ Get a mental picture of a relaxing place you know such as by the sea or in a garden
  - ○ Watch birds
  - ○ Think about a pleasant memory
  - ○ Talk things through with someone to get a more positive mental outlook and stop feeling overwhelmed with negative thoughts

Tip. Sometimes participants suggest using alcohol as a way of relaxing. While this is understandable, you may need to remind the group that even small amounts of alcohol can have a dramatic effect if their memory is already struggling.

Activity 4: relaxation exercise

There are many different types of relaxation and breathing exercises, and you may well have your own preferences. Often, people with dementia find a guided fantasy relaxation exercise easier than a muscle relaxation exercise in which they have to follow a set of instructions. If you do want to use an exercise that involves tensing, and then relaxing, different parts of the body, then before you start make sure that you know if any of the course participants have joint problems or an illness such as rheumatism which might make this difficult for them. If you have time, then you may want to try two different exercises and ask the group to choose which relaxation exercise they prefer.

Finally, remember to check that everyone in the group can hear you – this is especially important in this exercise as our voice often becomes quieter as we, ourselves, relax.

Either play a relaxation or breathing exercise (you may already have one that you like – and if not, then download one from the internet that you feel is suitable) or lead the group yourself with a relaxation exercise.

At the end of the exercise, make sure to find out whether participants have access to the internet or can find a relaxation or breathing exercise for themselves.

7 Session 4: finding a way through feelings

Session summary

Aim. In this session, we will continue to help participants to explore links between how dementia affects them, how they feel and how they cope. Many people living with dementia find that they cope best by learning to use words like "dementia" or "Alzheimer's disease" openly. However, others cope by avoiding them. For almost everyone, using these terms is often emotional, especially at first.

Context. Emotions play a large part in our lives and when coping with an illness such as dementia, the feelings people experience can be overwhelming. Helping the group to share with each other the feelings they experience can be critical in enabling the group to move forwards. Some people on the course are likely to be able to do this more easily than others. Now that the group has begun to form, participants may be starting to feel safer with each other and able to discuss their feelings more openly. For others in the course, however, doing this may be more difficult.

Process. A core issue that may prevent people from talking is what we refer to as "being in two minds" about dementia. This means that people with dementia may *both* feel as if they want to talk about their worries, for instance, about the future *and* at the same time be concerned that talking in this way will be upsetting for themselves or for those around them. Similarly, some people may feel not only both guilty and upset at not being able to drive or look after their finances, but also angry at being dependent on other people for help. There are many other potential examples of mixed feelings: upset, but determined to put a brave face on; frightened, but wanting to be in control; feeling embarrassed or stupid, but also worried that you're going mad. The key to this session is to help people to talk about all of these different emotions.

Content. This session focuses on anxiety and helping people to discuss their fears and uncertainties. Participants' emotional responses are the object of the session and the key activity for today is to give an opportunity for participants to explore their feelings together.

Table 7.1 Session plan for week four – finding a way through feelings

Objective	Activity	Duration	Resources	Expected outcome
To remind participants of last week's activity and help orient them to the purpose of this session.	Review	10 min	Last week's flip chart	Participants think and talk about aspects of their dementia.
To help participants identify their feelings about dementia.	How does dementia make you feel? Forgetful John (optional activity)	40 min	This handbook, flip chart and marker	Participants explore their feelings and think about sharing them with others.
To help participants consider the advantages and disadvantages of talking about their feelings.	Is it better not to talk about feelings?	40 min	This handbook, flip chart and marker	Participants realise that they can choose whether or not to discuss their feelings about dementia.

In the beginning, gently introduce the role of emotions in memory loss and living with dementia. Remember that not all participants will be able to talk about their emotions and other personal issues in the same way.

Activity 1: introduction and recap

Remind the group about the problems that have been identified in weeks one, two and three.

Activity 2: how does dementia make you feel?

The main focus of the course today is on encouraging participants to talk about how having a memory problem makes them feel. As a response to experiencing memory problems and dementia, people can go through a number of different emotions. Feeling worried, upset, angry or sad is common and is a natural reaction to a life-changing illness, such as dementia. Those feelings can be a first step in accepting the diagnosis and adjusting life so that people are able to live with dementia. However, sometimes participants will describe more extreme emotions: they may feel embarrassed or even ashamed. Sometimes people worry that they may be going mad and losing control – feelings which may be under-standable but which may stop them from coming to terms with the situation.

Ask people how they feel when they are reminded about their dementia – for instance, when they forget something or can't remember a name. Listen for the main emotions being expressed and write them up on a flip chart. Help participants to talk about the following:

✓ How they felt when they were first told about the possibility of dementia
✓ What they feel like now when they forget something
✓ Whether memory loss/dementia makes them feel angry, frustrated, sad, frightened about the future, anxious, embarrassed or stupid
✓ How they think other people respond if they realise a participant has a memory problem
✓ How they cope with this – for instance, do they avoid situations where they may forget something and feel embarrassed – such as going shopping?

Tip. Depending on how the group reacts, this might be a good opportunity to ask whether the group thinks that there is a stigma towards people with dementia. You might ask the group to discuss how society responded to famous peoples' diagnoses, such as Margaret Thatcher, Ronald Reagan, Terry Jones (from *Monty Python*) or Iris Murdoch – or the England World Cup winners of 1966 like Martin Peters, Nobby Stiles and Ray Wilson.

Look out for mention of these feelings and use prompts if appropriate:

✓ **Worry.** Ask participants how they feel when someone uses words like "dementia" and "Alzheimer's disease".
✓ **Grief.** Check with participants whether anyone feels as if they have lost something important if they find everyday tasks difficult. Perhaps this is a bit like a grieving process for them?
✓ **Frustration.** Ask people what the most frustrating thing is for them about memory loss/dementia. Is it the big things that change (for instance, not being able to drive) or the little things (for instance, forgetting where their glasses are) that have changed which are the worst?
✓ **Anger.** Do people in the course ever feel angry? If so, who are they most angry with – themselves or others? Can they be angry with the illness instead? Does the illness seem unfair?

Feelings about feelings. Sometimes participants will say that being worried or upset creates other feelings:

✓ **Embarrassment.** Watch out for people using expressions like "silly" or "stupid". If you hear this, then put this back to the group – check if others also feel embarrassed.
✓ **Guilt.** About being a burden to others, especially the people they love.
✓ **Going mad.** Did people worry that they were going mad, or that other people might look at them in this way?
✓ **Feeling overwhelmed or stuck.**

Tips.

✓ Listen out for what people are telling you. Listen for their actual words, as feelings are very subtle. Encourage people to clarify their feelings, but do not push them.

✓ Acknowledge the feelings within the group. Watch out for "group think" or the way in which one person assumes that they are speaking on behalf of the whole group.

✓ Remind the group that there are similarities and differences between participants – not everyone thinks in the same way.

✓ It's normal for groups to move towards and away from difficult feelings – try to gently encourage the group to talk about difficult issues that are brought up.

OPTIONAL ACTIVITY: FORGETFUL JOHN

If participants are struggling to talk about their own feelings towards dementia, then you may want to introduce this exercise as a way of prompting discussion. This is another fictional case: "Forgetful John".

I would now like to talk about someone who has problems remembering things. Let's call him John. Now John recently started losing things: for example, he often can't find his keys when going out for walk or to shop. At the weekend when his children came to visit, John couldn't remember the name of one of his grandchildren. John's wife and family have started to notice that he is forgetful, but nobody has talked to him about it yet.

Ask people to think about John, and how he may feel. Ask the group:

✓ *How do you think John feels about his memory problem?*
✓ *How might he feel when he forgets his grandson's name or loses his keys?*
✓ *Do you think he has anyone he can talk to about how he feels, for example his wife or a friend or his doctor?*
✓ *What do you think John might be worried about? Do you think he might be worried about having dementia or Alzheimer's disease?*

At the end of the "Forgetful John" exercise, ask the group if they have these feelings too – **importantly, ask the group if they, like John, worry about having dementia.**

Activity 3: is it better not to talk about feelings?

Discuss the pros and cons of talking about feelings. You can bring in the fictional character of John if you feel this is needed to prompt discussion.

We have talked about John, who's had some difficulties with remembering important things. We have also discussed how he might feel about this, and whether he might have talked to someone about how he feels. Perhaps John believes that it is better not to say anything – what are the advantages and disadvantages of this?

People might say things like, for example:

Advantages of not talking about feelings:

✓ It won't make things better
✓ It's upsetting for the person and their family to think about the possibility of dementia

Advantages of talking:

✓ John might be able to learn from other people
✓ It might help John to adjust – this way he will realise he's not alone
✓ Putting a name to something that you're worried about can make it seem less frightening
✓ Sharing experiences often makes people feel better – a problem shared is a problem halved

This discussion may bring up some difficult feelings for participants – so it is important to be aware of some symptoms of depression, as these can sometimes be missed:

✓ Changes in sleep
✓ Feeling hopeless
✓ Changes in appetite
✓ Losing temper more easily or crying
✓ Thoughts that life is not worth living

Finish up the session

At the end, distribute the handouts for this session and remind people to look at the handout at home with their partner. Ask the group how they would feel about telling people close to them about their feelings – do they think their family knows how they feel? **Importantly, make sure that participants know you are not telling them that they have to speak openly about how they feel – it's up to them what they do.**

8 Session 5: relationships – to tell or not to tell?

Session summary

Aim. This session focuses on social situations and relationships and the dilemma that people face in deciding whether to tell others that they have dementia. The aim of the session is not to tell people that they should disclose more – rather it is to encourage participants to think about the advantages and disadvantages of being more open about their dementia.

Context. While it may often be difficult for some people to do, telling others that you have dementia can bring advantages. Discussing difficult issues openly will often make communication clearer and will improve understanding on both sides. However, this can be a sensitive subject for participants to talk about as it can touch on deeply held fears that they will be looked down on. Sometimes people may feel that the best way to cope is to keep any difficulties that they may have to themselves.

Process. The important issue for the group is to discuss the advantages and disadvantages of disclosure openly, including being able to ask for help, so that participants can make their own decisions about whether to tell others.

Content. Central to today's session are two exercises, in which people will discuss the barriers to telling others about their dementia, and then the benefits of talking about this. Take the session at the pace at which participants feel comfortable talking. The session will also provide a chance to broaden the discussion to include issues around stigma and how society treats people with dementia.

Activity 1: introduction and reviewing previous week

Last week, we talked about the emotions you feel about having dementia. The focus for today's meeting is about whether you should tell other people about your dementia, and if so, what you say and who you say it to. This often brings up lots of issues for people: what does talking about dementia mean? What does it change? Can it help anything? We will discuss these questions today.

Table 8.1 Session plan for week five – relationships – to tell or not to tell?

Objective	Activity	Duration	Resources	Expected outcome
To recap week four.	Recap about coping with emotions	10 min	Last week's flip chart	The group will discuss how they have coped over the last week.
To encourage participants to think about how the dilemma of whether to tell others.	Telling participants about dementia	30 min	A flip chart and markers	Participants discuss the advantages and disadvantages of telling others.
To explore whether worrying about how others will react is a barrier to talking about dementia.	Reasons for telling and not telling people about it	20 min	A flip chart and markers	Participants discuss the risks and benefits of telling people about dementia.
To discuss ways to talk about dementia and ask others for help or to be more respectful.	Looking at participants' own examples	30 min	A flip chart, helpcards* and markers	Participants generate useful strategies for coping with their dementia in social situations and relationships.

* You can find "I have dementia" badges or helpcards at www.alzheimers.org.uk/info/20113/publications_about_living_with_dementia/774/helpcards.

However, before we do that, we will first remind ourselves what we discussed last week.

Remind the group about the previous week's discussions and ask the group specifically to talk about ways they have been coping with stress and emotions.

Activity 2: telling people about dementia

Distribute the handouts for this session to each person.

While one facilitator writes on the flip chart a list of the people that participants might tell, using Table 8.2 as a guide, the other facilitator asks participants if they talk to people about their dementia.

The first part of the activity involves suggesting the possibility to participants that even if they haven't explicitly told friends or relatives about their dementia, then many will have already guessed that something is wrong. If there are people with young-onset dementia, make sure their specific concerns are addressed, such as telling employees or teenage children about their dementia.

There are lots of reasons why it can be very difficult to talk about an illness like dementia. However, even if you haven't told someone that you have

Table 8.2 Who do you tell? (week five)

	I have already told them	I haven't told them, but they may suspect there is something wrong	I haven't told them, but they may need to know	I don't want to tell them
Husband/wife				
Adult children				
Siblings				
Grandchildren				
Close friends				
Employers/colleagues/ those I volunteer with				
Acquaintances				
People I meet (e.g. shop assistants)				
Others				

dementia, other people will often know that something has changed. We want to talk about this for a little while – let's think about who you have already talked about dementia with, and who you haven't told but might need to. Do you think that any one of these people might know anyway?

Activity 3: reasons for telling and not telling people about dementia

There's no right and wrong answer about who to tell, or whether you should tell anyone. But it's often helpful to think about what might help you to tell people or stop you from doing so.

Possible reasons for *not* telling. Ask people to discuss how other people might respond, for instance:

✓ Often people worry that others will think less of them if they know they have dementia.
✓ What do you think people will feel if you tell them that you have dementia?

Participants' possible responses may include:

☹ I will feel embarrassed.
☹ Other people won't be surprised.

49

☹ They will gossip about me – for instance, say that I'm "demented".

☹ I don't want to upset people. (NB: If people say this, follow it up – does it really mean "I don't want to upset myself?")

The barriers to talking about dementia are very understandable, and talking about dementia can sometimes be stressful and frightening. However, sharing problems and worries we have with other people can also be useful for various reasons.

Possible reasons for telling. Next, ask people to think about why they might want to tell others – how could it help them?

Participants' possible responses may include:

✓ They probably already knew but didn't know how to start a conversation with you.

✓ They probably knew something was wrong, but didn't know what it was – so telling people means that they don't get the wrong impression.

✓ It gives you more power and control over your life – being involved in making decisions.

Tip. Remember that it's not your job to tell people what to do – instead, get the group to think it through. There are no right or wrong answers. If participants say that they will tell other people, then ask them *what* they will tell. Often, people say different things to different people.

Activity 4: participants' own examples

Ask people to think about their experiences of talking to others about their dementia and asking other people for help or to change how they react.

* What have your experiences with GP, memory clinic or other professionals been like?
* Have you ever had any problems when you can't work out the right change in a shop, or if you forget where you left your car or if you need help to find the toilet? If so, then how do you explain this to people?
* How would you feel about wearing an "I have dementia" badge?
* How would you feel about carrying a helpcard?
* Do you feel you can ask people to slow down or explain things again?

Use the handout to discuss these and the group's other examples of interactions that may occur in social situations.

Look at things that other people do that are helpful and unhelpful (draw a line down the flip chart with helpful on one side and unhelpful on the other side).

Discuss the different ways in which you can ask for help.

9 Session 6: what is dementia?

Aim. This session provides an opportunity for participants to discuss their experiences of living with dementia and to ask you any questions that they might have about their illness. The session, therefore, combines information giving with short discussions about the particular topics.

Context. Now that we have helped people to talk about their worries about dementia, the group will be strong enough to talk in more depth about dementia and the different types of this syndrome.

Process and Content. Before the start of this session, make sure that you know what diagnosis each of the different participants has been given, where they received their diagnosis and when this happened. You may need to use this information to prompt participants (although be careful not to reveal any confidential information). The session will focus on the symptoms and diagnostic process of the two main types of dementia, but if some participants have other diagnoses, then you will need to have information to hand out about these as well. In the activities, you should encourage participants to talk about what it was like to get a diagnosis, their experiences after this of living with dementia and the different symptoms they might have now.

Activity 1: introduction and reminder of the last week's topic

Use the previous week's flip chart and ask participants to talk about:

- Which (if any) strategies they used to cope in the past week
- Which strategies they found helpful
- Whether they talked about dementia to anyone and how it made them feel

Today we will talk a little more about dementia and what different types there are. We will first discuss what you know about dementia and what you would like to know, to make sure that your questions are answered. Then, we will talk

Table 9.1 Session plan for week six – what is dementia?

Objective	Activity	Duration	Resources	Expected outcome
To remind participants about the previous week.	Reminder of the last week's topic	5 min	Last week's flip chart	Participants are able to make a connection with the previous week's work.
To introduce dementia as a topic and establish baseline level of knowledge.	What does the group know about . . . ?	15 min	Flip chart and marker	Participants warm up to this week's topic and to think about what they already know about dementia.
To introduce idea of a dementia journey.	The dementia journey	20 min	Flip chart, marker and handouts	Participants integrate different elements of their experiences.
To gain a better understanding about dementia.	What is dementia?	20 min	Flip chart, marker and handouts	Participants have a better understanding about the illness and its effects.
To gain a better understanding of the different types of dementia and their treatment.	Different types of dementia	20 min	Flip chart, marker and handouts	Participants have a better understanding of different types of dementia, including their own and its treatment.
To introduce the idea of the future and care options.	The journey after diagnosis	10 min	Handouts and local knowledge	Participants have a better understanding of follow-up and future care for themselves and their relatives and friends.

about the different types of dementia, its treatment and what you can do to help yourselves.

Activity 2: what does the group know about dementia?

Go around the group and ask participants to describe:

- ✓ Whether they remember being diagnosed with dementia
- ✓ What their individual diagnosis was (e.g. Alzheimer's disease, vascular dementia, frontal dementia, Lewy body dementia)
- ✓ What they already know about dementia and whether there is anything they would like to learn

The purpose of this activity is to establish what participants' knowledge is about their diagnosis and to gauge their feelings about this. Where participants are curious about their diagnosis, you can make sure that you spend enough time discussing that particular information later on. On the other hand, if you see that participants are wary about an issue, then you can talk about it in a more cautious way.

Distribute the handouts for this session. Briefly describe the way in which future sessions will address what people can do, and what support there is available, but don't go into any of these in great detail at this point.

Activity 3: the dementia journey

Sometimes people use the phrase "dementia journey" to describe what happens to someone, from when they first suspect there is something wrong with their memory, all the way through their assessment and illness.

For most people, the first station or stop on the dementia journey is with their GP. As many people here will know from experience, if a doctor thinks that a person might have dementia, then they will do a number of tests to find out how a person's memory is functioning, and whether any of their problems can be explained by another illness. The tests can also help determine which type of dementia people have:

✓ *Taking medical history. The first part of the assessment is to identify whether other conditions such as depression, psychosis or Parkinson's disease might explain your problems.*
✓ *Tests of memory. You may have been asked questions to see how well you can remember (for instance, you may have been asked to spell the word "world" backward or to take seven away from 100). These tests (sometimes called cognitive tests) give an idea of how well your memory is working.*
✓ *Head scan. Often, patients are asked to have a head scan – a type of x-ray of the brain – in the hospital. This will likely to show whether there are any visible changes in the brain.*
✓ *Blood and urine tests. These are usually done to screen for alternative causes of memory problems, for example, an infection.*

Where do people get their diagnosis? For some people, it is just their GP that they see, but for most people, the next stop on the journey is a specialist doctor in a memory clinic.

As you go through the handouts, write up on the flip-chart people's responses to these issues:

✓ What was their experience of being given the different tests? How did the whole experience make them feel?
✓ How were they given the diagnosis?
✓ How did this make them feel?
✓ What happened afterwards?

Activity 4: what is dementia?

"Dementia" is a word that is used to describe a group of different illnesses, all of which are alike and have similar symptoms. (If dementia is diagnosed before the age of 65 it is called young-onset dementia.) The most common of

these illnesses are Alzheimer's disease and vascular dementia, but there are also many more. As well as differences between the illnesses, there are also differences in how individuals experience the same types of dementia. However, most people will have some or all of these symptoms:

- ✓ **Memory loss**, *particularly of recent events. This may not be severe at first, but it is likely to become progressively worse.*
- ✓ *Problems **finding the right words** for what you want to say.*
- ✓ *Feeling **disoriented**. For example, not recognising familiar streets and becoming confused about the time of day.*
- ✓ *Having trouble **thinking clearly** and **doing practical tasks** that you used to do easily.*
- ✓ *Problems with **mobility** or **balance** or **visual perception** .*
- ✓ **Changes in behaviour** *– but this may be a reaction to the dementia such as sense of insecurity.*

Ask people to discuss with the group:

- ✓ How do people experience their own symptoms?
- ✓ Which symptoms do people feel they have?

Activity 5: different types of dementia

The two most common types of dementia are Alzheimer's disease and vascular dementia. We will now briefly talk about each of them.

Alzheimer's disease

What is Alzheimer's disease? *Alzheimer's disease is caused by damage to the nerve cells in the brain. The pattern of damage can vary between individuals, so that the difficulties experienced by one person will not be exactly the same as the next. It is the most common type of dementia.*

What causes Alzheimer's disease? *Although there are many theories as to why this disease happens, we still don't know what causes it, other than that it is more common with age.*

Is it something that can be passed on to your children? *There is an inherited form of the disease, but this is rare. Only in a very small number of highly unusual cases, which occur early in life, is Alzheimer's disease passed from one generation to the next.*

Is there any treatment? *There is no cure for Alzheimer's disease. However, some people are able to have medication that can help with some of the problems of a poor memory. The most common of these is called Aricept. We also know that it is important for people with Alzheimer's disease to stay as active as possible – to stay physically fit, to have as many friends and social outlets as possible and to find ways to stimulate themselves mentally.*

Does it become worse? *Yes, but the speed at which Alzheimer's disease becomes worse can vary – for many people, the illness progresses quite slowly. Research is now looking at whether there may be things you can do to slow it down.*

Vascular dementia

What is vascular dementia? *This is caused by blockages or bleeding within the brain. This is often linked with heart disease and has the same risk factors – such as high blood pressure and high levels of cholesterol. After Alzheimer's disease, vascular dementia is the next most common form of dementia. Moreover, many people have a mixed form of both illnesses.*

Can vascular dementia be passed on? *This can happen, but only in the way that risks for heart disease in general can be passed on. Recent research suggests that the factors that make vascular dementia more likely are also risks factors of Alzheimer's disease.*

Is there any treatment? *There are no cures for vascular dementia. Unlike Alzheimer's disease, Aricept cannot be prescribed for people with vascular dementia. However, aspirin is often suggested, as this helps to prevent strokes from happening. There are also other things that you can do to try to reduce the speed at which the dementia will become worse:*

- *Make sure you keep your blood pressure under control.*
- *If you smoke, then try to stop or cut down.*
- *If you drink alcohol, then make sure you drink in moderation.*
- *If you are a diabetic, then make sure you keep this under control.*
- *Make sure you take a good amount of exercise.*
- *Eat a healthful diet.*
- *Maintain social contact and hobbies as far as possible.*

If you have people in the group with other forms of dementia such as Lewy body dementia, make sure you include information about this. You may wish to give some additional information with the handout for this session.

As well as helping participants to discuss their illness, this is also a chance to get people to discuss their fears about the future if they wish. While talking about the future is a difficult issue, it may be an important worry for some people. They might benefit from seeing that others in the group who may have more severe problems can still live with them and manage their situation.

Activity 6: the journey after diagnosis

In addition to family and friends, emotional and practical support is available from a range of services, including voluntary organisations and health and social care. Try to think of local examples to tell the group about (and if you have people with young-onset dementia, look for examples tailored to them), but remind them that you will come back to this issue later on.

Ask people to discuss whether they have been in contact with any support groups. What do people think about the support they might have received?

10 Session 7: living as well as you can

Session summary

Aim. The aim of this session is to look at the practical things people can do to ensure that they live well with dementia.

Context. We will build on previous weeks in suggesting that people with dementia can take an active role in making decisions about their life.

Process. This is often a delicate subject to talk about, as it involves facing a future in which abilities that people have now may gradually disappear. The linking theme within the session is around the possibility of actively looking to take control of one's life – either by making a decision to do more of the things that you enjoy or by planning ahead.

Content. The key method used today will be group discussions, through which you will try to help people think about different issues that might be new to them. You will also encourage people to explore their own thoughts about what they can do to live well and to adjust to their situation. Some of the topics today will be more difficult, for example, talking about the future and thinking how people can adjust to it.

Table 10.1 Session plan for week seven – living as well as you can

Objective	Activity	Duration	Resources	Expected outcome
To go over work from the previous week.	Recap of the last session	10 min	Previous flip charts	This is a reminder of the previous topic and a starting point for today's session.
To help participants to think about the things they can do to have control.	What can people do well?	40 min	Flip chart and marker	Participants realise what makes them feel good or positive and identify areas in which they can take control of their life.
To introduce Advanced Care Planning and think about driving.	Taking charge of your life and driving	40 min	Flip chart, marker and handouts	Participants discuss different elements of Advanced Care Planning and issues around driving.

Activity 1: introduction and recap

Today we will talk about how you can live well with dementia. This means understanding how dementia affects you, recognising how you feel about it and how this affects what you do and don't do. Once you know more about this, we will discuss what changes you might be able to make and how to go about them. The aim will be to help you feel more confident about yourselves.

Tip. If there are people with young-onset dementia, people who are still working, or both, ensure you address this in the discussion.

Remind the group about the previous week – ask participants if:

✓ They found talking about the diagnosis of dementia last week difficult.
✓ They have talked to anyone else about dementia.
✓ How did this make people feel?

Activity 2: what can people do well?

It is important to recognise the things that you are good at and that are going well. Knowing what you are good at can help you to feel good about yourselves and also help you to feel more confident. We will now look at the things that you feel good about, that are meaningful for you or that are going well for you.
Ask course participants to name one thing that is going well for them at the moment, including things that they would like to do more of, that give them a sense of hope or purpose or that they feel positive about.

Write the ideas on the flip chart so people can see it written up. You can use these positive things to help people reflect on how they feel in such situations. Do people feel positive, relaxed, confident, and so forth when things go well?

Tip. Help participants find at least one positive thing. Ask open questions and use your own observations and knowledge of them to help them with this if they feel stuck or are negative.

Taking on new challenges

It is often important to have new challenges in life – this can give you a new way to look at life and that might help you to feel better. Perhaps you could try:

* *Taking things up that you haven't done for a while (which may perhaps need to be done in a different way).*
* *Picking up a hobby or attending a club.*
* *Thinking about doing mental exercises such as crosswords or quizzes on TV.*
* *Having a healthy lifestyle – getting exercise and having a good diet (we will talk about this more next week)*

- *Asking yourself how you have coped with difficult times in the past. Are there things that helped you then that you think could help you now?*

Activity 3: taking charge of your life – Advanced Care Planning

In previous weeks, we discussed the way in which some people talk about a "dementia journey". Part of this journey involves thinking about the future – something that is often very difficult for people to do, as it means acknowledging that things may get worse. However, some people find it helpful to feel that they have made decisions about their future. Often, this is something that a person can do, and then forget about – safe in the knowledge that if things become worse, then they have made preparations.

Amongst the ways in which you could take charge of your life are:

- ❖ *Talking to people around you about the future*
- ❖ *Making a lasting power of attorney*
- ❖ *Making a will*
- ❖ *Making a "living will" (advance decisions and advance statements)*

Lasting power of attorney and advance statements

A lasting power of attorney (LPA) is one of a number of ways to plan ahead. Other ways to plan ahead are advance statements or advance decisions. These allow you to put in writing that you want to refuse certain treatments, or your preferences about other care choices.

An LPA lets you choose a person you trust to act for you if you come to a point where you can't make decisions yourself. This person is referred to as your "attorney", and you can choose what decisions they are allowed to make for you.

One type of LPA covers decisions about your property and finances, while the other covers decisions about your health and welfare. You can choose to designate both types or just one. You can appoint the same person to make both types of decisions for you, or you can ask different people to do each of them.

If you want to create an LPA, then there are forms you need to complete before they are registered – these are available on the internet, or the Alzheimer's Society can provide you with information about this.

Other things you might think about are putting your finances in order and making (or updating) your will.

Ask the group to think about what else people can do to take charge of their lives. Would setting goals to do hobbies and activities help people feel more confident?

Activity 4: driving

Not being able to drive is one of the biggest issues that many people with dementia face. But having a diagnosis of dementia is not in itself necessarily a reason to stop driving. What matters, from both a legal and a practical point of view, is whether you are still able to drive safely.

However, if you have been given a diagnosis of dementia and you want to continue to drive, then you must do two things:

First, by law, you must inform the Driver and Vehicle Licensing Agency (DVLA). The DVLA will ask you for your permission for them to contact your GP and/or specialists (such as the memory clinic). On the basis of the information they get back from the doctors, they will make a decision as to whether you can continue to drive. They may also ask you to take a driving test.

Second, you must also immediately inform your car insurance company. If you don't, then your policy may become invalid.

Although giving up driving is often hard, there are many ways around the problems that stopping driving can create – for instance, the money that you save will often more than cover the cost of getting a taxi or bus more regularly. Let's talk about this for a while.

Ask the group:

- ✓ Who still drives?
- ✓ Who has given up because of their diagnosis?
- ✓ What were the effects of this?
- ✓ What can they do instead of driving to places?
- ✓ How do they feel about the different alternatives?

Try to help people think of other options available for travelling and encourage them to discuss this in the group. Dementia may be a condition that qualifies people for a blue badge – it is up to local councils, so check your area.

Finish up the session

One way to finish the session is with a quote from James McKillop. Use this to summarise what people have said and to prompt more thought at this point. Finally, remind people to work on the handout with their partners at home.

To finish up today's session, I am going to read two sentences from a Scottish man who had been diagnosed with dementia – James McKillop. He wrote these ideas down a couple of years after receiving his diagnosis. James became a well-known figure in Scotland, advocating for the rights of people with dementia.

Being told I had dementia was like a door re-opening after a difficult time in my life – new challenges, new opportunities.

I want people to understand that dementia isn't an end, it's a new beginning where you do things differently. While some things change forever there is a lot you still can do.

James McKillop (2003)

11   Session 8: staying active

Session summary

Aim. This session has two aims: first, to continue to address issues around participants being active and taking control of their life, and second, to act as a final review session in which you can say goodbye to members of the course.

Context. While there is a final, post-group session with relatives and partners next week, this is the last chance you have to say goodbye to this group.

Process and Content. As this is the final session, you should help the group to think about the end of the group meetings, and what people can do to live as actively as possible in the future. Use this last group session to say goodbye. You can discuss what people thought about what they have learnt and what they remember. You may want to think about having a celebration at the end of the group – for instance, by bringing in a cake or finding another way to mark the achievement. Today will involve review about the past sessions and discussions about people's plans for their future. We will focus on how people can use what they have learnt in the sessions and how they can stay active and take control.

Activity 1: introduction and recap

Today we will talk about how we can stay active and continue to live actively. We will talk about what you remember the most from the session and if there are other things you would like to find out. This is the last session where all the participants have a diagnosis of dementia. We have come a long way and worked hard to get here and learn about dementia and living with it. So we all deserve a small celebration. (Distribute handouts at this point.)

In order to check participants' progress, remind them briefly about any goals they may have made at the start of the course – as well as the different forms of Advanced Care Planning that you discussed last week. Check whether they have discussed this with their families – and whether they plan to act on any of them, and if not, then what stops them from doing it?

Table 11.1 Session plan for week eight – staying active

Objective	Activity	Duration	Resources	Expected outcome
To discuss the previous session and progress since then.	Introduction and recap of the previous session	10 min	Previous flip charts	Participants are reminded about what they did last week and discuss making active decisions.
To focus on activities that maintain health and well-being.	What can you do to stay active?	25 min	Flip chart, marker and handouts	People think about what they can do to stay active and why it is beneficial for them.
To reflect on progress, changes and what still needs to be covered.	Review of what has been covered	25 min	Flip charts from all previous sessions	Participants are helped to reflect on changes that have occurred.
To think about what the important elements of the sessions are that need to be fed back to relatives and friends.	What to talk about with family and friends?	20 min	Flip charts from all previous sessions	Participants agree what needs to be discussed (or not discussed) in the meeting with relatives and friends.
To find the words to say goodbye to each participant.	Saying goodbye	10 min		Participants will feel valued and heard by course facilitators.

You might want to think if there are ways to celebrate the end of the course and congratulate participants for their efforts – for instance, by bringing a cake or biscuits.

Activity 2: what can you do to stay active?

We are now going to talk about different ways in which you can be active. You have already been working hard to find ways to live well with dementia and to adapt to the changes it brings. Let's now talk about the most important things that we discussed in the sessions, and what you can do to benefit from them even when the group has finished.

Last week, we talked about how you can live well. Let's now discuss what exactly you can do to stay active. What can you do to feel good physically and mentally?

To feel good, you need to focus on both physical and mental well-being. This involves physical activity, mental activity, social activity and also a good diet.

Physical activity

Evidence shows that regular exercise helps people to stay well for longer. Being physically active also helps to prevent depression and helps you feel well. You could take a short walk for 20 minutes every day or play with grandchildren or exercise your upper body when sitting down.

If you smoke, then try to cut this down.

Mental activity

Keep your brain and mind active by doing various exercises and having fun playing games. This can, in turn, help you feel more confident and able. You could, for example:

❖ *Read the newspaper/magazines*
❖ *Work on jigsaw puzzles*
❖ *Solve crossword puzzles and sudoku*
❖ *Play card or board games with your friends or family*
❖ *Find something to do every day that you feel good at*
❖ *Find something to do every day that you enjoy*

Social activity

Research shows that people who are sociable and have lots of contact with other people are happier. Keeping in touch with close friends and family regularly can also help your mind be active. This will, again, be beneficial to your well-being, confidence and abilities. You could, for example:

• *Have a cup of tea or coffee with family, friends, neighbours or your church group if that is where you go*
• *Go to local support groups*
• *Go shopping and do other activities outside the home with other people*
• *Meet new people*

Diet and nutrition

What we eat is important for how we feel. Good food also helps the body and the brain to work efficiently, so make sure you have enough of the good stuff.

• *Eat five portions of fruit and vegetables every day.*
• *Eat "good" fat, such as oily fish and avocado, and less "bad" fat, such as red meat.*

Many people find that having a regular routine and having a structure to the day means that they can do these things consistently.

Ask people to talk about how they feel about the different activities. What else can they do for themselves? How can they keep doing the activities?

Activity 3: review of what has been covered so far

Briefly go over the eight weeks of the course – use the flip charts to remind people about what has been covered. Ask participants:

✓ What are the most important things they took from the group?
✓ Which of the topics covered have people looked to apply?

Encourage participants to talk about the questions and say something, however insignificant it may seem. Praising even small steps will be a support for them to do more in the future. Help people to focus on the benefits and write them up on a flip chart to aid the process.

Activity 4: what to talk about with family and/or friends?

Remind people that the next week's session will be different, as family and friends will be present and it will be the final session. There may have been issues that came up in the course that participants do want to talk about or do not want to talk about – so now is the time to talk about those issues. Ask participants:

✓ Are there any issues people find it difficult to discuss with their family and friends? If so, what are they?
✓ What would they like to talk about with their family and friends next week?

This will help you not only plan the next session, but also help people think about the end, and finally to think about sharing with partners.

Activity 5: saying goodbye

Saying goodbye involves being sad. Some participants may be more aware of this than others. Allow people in the group to feel sad if they need to do so. Some participants might want to keep meeting outside of the structured sessions. If they do this, then ideally, it is best if the whole group is involved – otherwise, some participants may feel distressed at being excluded. Ask participants:

✓ How do they feel about the end of the group?
✓ How are they going to cope with the end?

As the final activity, each of you – the facilitators – should go around the group and say a personalised "goodbye" to each participant. You may want to thank each participant for one thing they brought to the group, or tell each person one way in which you will remember them.
    This is likely to be a good point for the group to end.

12 Post-group session: bringing it all together

Aim. This is the final session for participants and their partners or family members. The main aims of the session are to review what has been achieved over the course of the sessions and to think ahead.

Context. This session provides a good opportunity for participants and partners to give feedback about any changes, benefits or less good things that have happened as a result of the sessions. Partners in particular will need space to articulate their concerns – but this needs to be framed as a commentary, rather than as the main substance of the course – about what has occurred within the sessions. Also use this session to allow the group to say their goodbyes and to talk about things participants can do after the group – for instance, to draw on the other support that there is in your area.

Process and Content. Before the session, make sure that you know about all the other support services that are available in your area and have as many leaflets and information ready to distribute as possible. You will also need the flip charts from all sessions to act as prompts for what was discussed and what the participants have gained (remember to be guided by discussion on this in the previous session). You may not need all of the 90 minutes for this session. Feel free to be explicit about what the group meant to you personally and what you have learnt or gained. Finally, remember to thank everyone in the group for their contribution.

Activity 1: review of all previous sessions

Have all the flip charts from the course ready to use and refer to. Before the session, put them in the order that they were created during the sessions. Starting with the first meeting you had with the group, put the flip charts up for people to see. Briefly remind them what was discussed and then give participants and their partners an opportunity to give feedback and talk about:

Table 12.1 Session plan for the post-group session – bringing it all together

Objective	Activity	Duration	Resources	Expected outcome
To review the course as a whole – reinforcing both the overall message of the course and of each session.	Review of all sessions	40 min	All relevant flip charts from previous sessions	Participants and partners are reminded of the key issues, and to discuss how they applied them.
To plan ahead and remind people what support is available locally.	Further support	20 min	Information about local support options	Participants will be more aware of what they can do after the sessions.
To allow partners and participants to reflect on what the group has meant for them.	Saying goodbye	30 min	Certificate of attendance (optional)	Participants and their families share their thoughts about the course.

✓ What they remember about the session and their feelings about this
✓ Whether they have been able to apply in real life what they learnt
✓ Their partner's views about the sessions

In particular, address the information from the preliminary and first week, so that participants can reflect on their hopes, fears and expectations from the start of the course – this will enable participants to reflect on what has been achieved and what has still to be addressed.

Activity 2: further support

In advance of the session, gather as much information as you can about other local support groups and services that participants can draw on. Have these available for people if they want them. Although you might have discussed this in the previous session, bringing the topic up again with partners present will help people to address their anxieties over the ending of the group.

Rather than simply giving advice, you can ask people to discuss what opportunities for support and local activities they are aware of.

❖ Ask participants and their partners to share their ideas about what is available.
❖ Encourage discussion about participants meeting after the sessions.

Activity 3: saying goodbye

After discussing the sessions with participants and their partners, it's time to say goodbye.

There are many different ways to do this – either you can speak first, or you can ask participants and their partners to speak first. You should give everyone present an opportunity to reflect on their experiences and to comment both on what has been achieved and what remains to be faced. Many facilitators like to finish the session by thanking everyone who has come individually for their contribution, finding one positive thing to say about each person.

In some sense, this repeats the goodbye that was said at the end of the previous session – however, that is not necessarily a bad thing, as it allows you to thank people for their unique contribution in front of their partner – and also to thank their partner for their work. You might also think about other ways of marking or celebrating participants' achievements – for instance, by presenting participants with a certificate of attendance.

(NB: There are no handouts for this session other than the information that you will bring about other sources of support available locally.)

Further reading

Bender, M. (2004) *Therapeutic Groupwork for People with Cognitive Losses: Working with People with Dementia*. Bicester, UK: Speechmark Publishing Ltd.

Cheston, R. (1996) Stories and Metaphors: Talking about the Past in a Psychotherapy Group for People with Dementia, *Ageing and Society*, 16, 579–602.

Cheston, R. (2013) Dementia as a Problematic Experience: Using the Assimilation Model as a Framework for Psychotherapeutic Work with People with Dementia, *Neurodisability and Psychotherapy*, 1 (1), 70–95.

Cheston, R. (2015) The Role of the Fear-of-Loss-of-Control Marker within the Accounts of People Affected by Dementia about Their Illness: Implications for Psychotherapy, *Quaderni di Psicoterapia Cognitiva*, 37, 45–66, doi: 10.3280/qpc2015-037003.

Cheston, R. and Bender, M. (1999) *Understanding Dementia: The Man with the Worried Eyes*. London: Jessica Kingsley Publishers Ltd.

Cheston, R., Gatting, L., Marshall, A., Spreadbury, J. and Coleman, P. (2017) Markers of Assimilation of Problematic Experiences in Dementia within the LIVDEM Project, *Dementia: The International Journal of Social Research and Policy*, 16 (4), 443–460, doi: 10.1177/1471301215602473.

Cheston, R. and Howells, L. (2015) A Feasibility Study of Translating "Living Well with Dementia" Groups into a Primary Care IAPT Service (Innovative Practice), *Dementia: The International Journal of Social Research and Policy*, published on-line 17 April, doi: 10.1177/1471301215582104.

Cheston, R. and Ivanecka, A. (2017) Individual and Group Psychotherapy with People Affected by Dementia: A Systematic Review of the Literature, *International Journal of Geriatric Psychiatry*, 32 (1), 3–31, doi: 10.1002/gps.4529.

Cheston, R., Jones, K. and Gilliard, J. (2003) Group Psychotherapy and People with Dementia, *Aging and Mental Health*, 7 (6), 452–461.

Cheston, R. and Jones, R. (2009) A Small-Scale Study Comparing the Impact of Psycho-Education and Exploratory Psychotherapy

Groups on Newcomers to a Group for People with Dementia, *Aging and Mental Health*, 13 (3), 410–425.

Cheston, R., Marshall, A., Jones, A., Spreadbury, J. and Coleman, P. (2018) Living Well with Dementia Groups: Changes in Participant and Therapist Verbal Behaviour, *Aging and Mental Health*, 22 (1), 61–69, doi: 10.1080/13607863.2016.1231171.

Folstein, M., Folstein, S. and McHugh, P. (1975) "Mini-Mental State": A Practical Method for Grading the Cognitive State of Patients for the Clinician, *Journal of Psychiatric Research*, 12, 189–198.

Logsdon, R., Pike, K.C., McCurry, S.M., Hunter, P., Maher, J., Snyder, L. and Teri, L. (2010) Early-Stage Memory Loss Support Groups: Outcomes from a Randomized Controlled Clinical Trial, *The Journals of Gerontology, Series B. Psychological Sciences and Social Sciences*, November, 65B (6), 691–697.

Marshall, A. (2004) Coping in Early Dementia: Findings of a New Type of Support Group. In B. Miesen and G. Jones (Eds.), *Care-Giving in Dementia: Research and Applications*, Volume 3. London: Routledge.

Marshall, A., Spreadbury, J., Cheston, R., Coleman, P., Ballinger, C., Mullee, M., Pritchard, J., Russell, C. and Bartlett, E. (2015) A Pilot Randomised Control Trial to Compare Changes in Quality of Life for Participants with Early Diagnosis Dementia Who Attend a "Living Well with Dementia" Group Compared to Waiting List Control, *Aging and Mental Health*, 19 (6), 526–535, doi: 10.1080/13607863.2014.954527.

McKillop, J. (2003) *Opening Shutters-Opening Minds*. Dementia Services Development Centre, Stirling: University of Stirling.

Moniz-Cook, E. and Manthorpe, J. (2009) Personalising Psychosocial Interventions to Person Needs and Context. In E. Moniz-Cook and J. Manthorpe (Eds.), *Early Psychosocial Interventions in Dementia*. London: Jessica Kingsley Publishers Ltd.

Preston, L., Bucks, R.S. and Marshall, A. (2005) Investigating the Ways That Older People Cope with Dementia: The Role of Identity, *BPS Special Interest Group for the Elderly Newsletter*, 90, 8–14.

Watkins, R., Cheston, R., Jones, K. and Gilliard, J. (2006) "Coming Out" with Alzheimer's Disease: Changes in Awareness during a Psychotherapy Group for People with Dementia, *Aging and Mental Health*, 10, 166–176.

Appendix: handouts for sessions

The following handouts can be downloaded from the eResources:
www.routledge.com/9781138542358

PRELIMINARY SESSION HANDOUT: PRELIMINARY MEETING FOR PARTICIPANTS AND PARTNERS

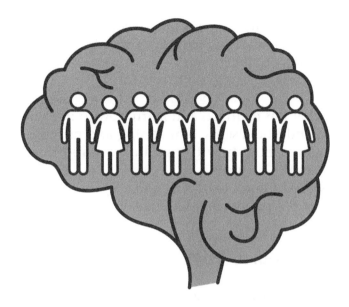

This session is to introduce the *Living Well with Dementia* course and to help you and your family or friends to learn about what coming to the sessions will involve.

Dementia is often a difficult subject to discuss.

However, many people with dementia benefit from talking about what is happening to them. This course provides people with a safe place to meet and talk to others who are going through the same experiences as they are and to learn more about the challenges that they face.

What will you get out of coming to the course?

✓ You will meet other people with memory problems.
✓ You will learn more about memory loss and how to cope with any problems that come up.
✓ You will have a chance to talk through any difficulties you have with people who understand what it's like.

We will try and give everyone who comes a chance to talk about their problems, but you will not have to talk about anything that you don't feel comfortable doing.

What do we mean by "living well with dementia"?

In these groups, we will focus on "living well" with dementia. What we mean by this is that we want to help you and your family to live as fulfilling a life as you can despite any difficulties that you might face.

Talking with other people who are going through similar experiences is important because that way we learn that we're not alone. But this is also difficult – sometimes it's only natural to want to forget about difficult things.

In the course we will talk at times about "living well", but we know that there is no cure for dementia. So you cannot recover in the sense of getting better. Coming to the course won't help you to have a better memory, but we hope that you will be more able to find a way to improve your quality of life – to live better.

We believe the best way to do this is to:

✓ Adjust to what has changed and learn how to live with it.
✓ Be hopeful and find a sense of meaning and purpose in life.
✓ Make decisions about how things are now and how you would like them to be in the future.
✓ Find a way around problems that come up.
✓ Feel a part of life rather than feeling shut out of it.

How long will the course last?

The course will take place once every week for eight weeks. Each meeting will last 90 minutes – and we would suggest that you aim to come to the groups 10 minutes or so before they start to give you a chance to prepare and to meet socially.

What will we be doing in the sessions?

Each of our sessions will cover a specific theme. The sessions are often linked, so that most themes will be covered in two or more sessions.

Week number	Key theme
Preliminary meeting	Welcome and Introductions (with partners)
Week one	Is there anything wrong with me?
Week two	Memory aids and strategies
Week three	Worry, stress and memory
Week four	Finding a way through feelings
Week five	To tell or not to tell?
Week six	What is dementia?
Weeks seven	Living as well as you can with dementia
Week eight	Staying active
Post-group	Bringing it all together (with partners)

Each week, you will be given an information sheet that you can add into your folder. It is important that you read through the handouts at home with your partner. Talk to your partner about the handouts and try the exercises. They should help you feel more relaxed and develop effective ways of reminding yourself of the important things. Talking about the groups and doing the exercises at home will also help you benefit from the sessions.

Is there anyone I can contact to discuss the course with?

People sometimes have doubts about whether the course is for them. However, our experience is that if they stick with it, then by the end of the eight weeks almost everyone is glad that they came.

If you do have concerns about coming to the course, then please contact your local organisers.

Fill in the names and contact numbers for your course leader and any other important people at this group below:

_____

_____

_____

_____

_____

_____

_____

_____

WEEK ONE HANDOUT: IS THERE ANYTHING WRONG WITH ME?

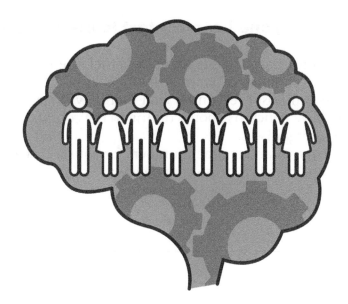

The main theme of today has been to identify things that people on the course struggle with, and things that are going better. It may be your memory that isn't working well, or it may be something else, like using words and names. You may also be struggling with some skills that you've taken for granted – like driving or going shopping.

On the other hand, there may well be many other things in your life that you are doing just as well now as you ever have.

Take a few minutes to make a list of each of them.

Things I do well	Problems I experience

WEEK TWO HANDOUT: MEMORY AIDS AND STRATEGIES

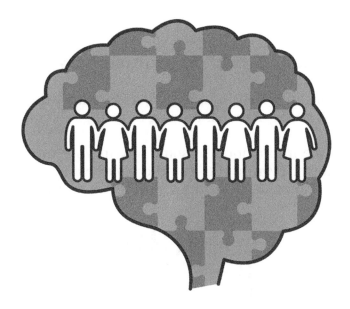

How does memory work?

One way to think about memory is to distinguish between immediate memory, which holds the information that we see or hear for a few seconds, and long-term memory, in which we store information so that we can remember it the next day, the next week or the next year.

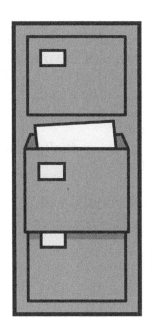

Make sure the information goes into your memory

As we get older, and particularly if we have problems with our memory, so our long-term memory becomes less effective. We, therefore, have to make more of an effort to make sure that information goes into our long-term memory.

How to make things "stick" in your memory

In order to remember new information, it helps if we do something with it in our mind rather than just hearing or seeing it. For instance:

✓ Organise the information in some way in your mind. For example, write it down. Even if you lose the paper, you will still have more chance of making it stick through the act of writing.

✓ Make a link between the new information and something familiar you already know. For example, if you meet someone called Peter, you might make the link "Peter Pan" if he looks young.
✓ A letter of the alphabet can be a cue – so "P" for "Pea" if Peter has a round face. Once you have the first letter of a name, it acts as a trigger to help you remember it.
✓ Repeat it to yourself – but gradually making the gaps between the repetitions longer and longer.

Getting it right the first time around will help to reduce mistakes later on.

Memory aids

It is important to use a diary, calendar or notebook to help you to remember what you need. Writing out the day's events on a white board that you can clean off and renew is another excellent way to help your memory. Sometimes a simple change such as making sure that any glasses or hearing aids that you use work properly can make a great difference.

Do you have any suggestions as to how to help improve your memory?

Here is a space for you to list any ways of improving your memory that you think you would find useful:

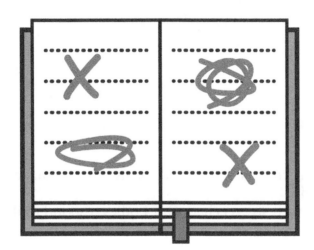

1 _____

2 _____

3 _____

4 _____

5 _____

WEEK THREE HANDOUT: WORRY, STRESS AND MEMORY

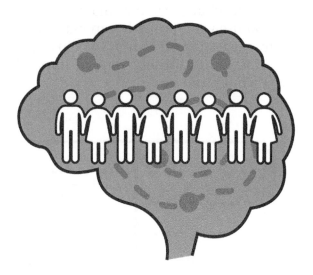

A little bit of stress is often good for us – it can make us feel energised and focussed.

But too much stress is bad. Our bodies respond as if we are in danger or under threat:

☹ Our muscles become tense
☹ Our breathing rate increases
☹ Our heart beats faster
☹ When this happens, it is hard to concentrate or to think clearly
☹ This means it is harder to remember things that happen

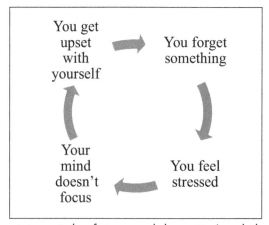

The vicious circle of stress and dementia (week three)

Coping with the physical symptoms of stress

It is helpful to recognise when you are starting to get stressed and learn ways to cope with it.

If you can't remember things, try to tell yourself it doesn't matter and it will probably come back later. Getting worked up will just make it worse.

Try and distract yourself as a way of relaxing

- ✓ Listen to music
- ✓ Look at things around you and try to focus on what is happening
- ✓ Get a mental picture of a relaxing place you know such as by the sea or in a garden
- ✓ Watch birds
- ✓ Think about a pleasant memory

Often, people use alcohol as a way of relaxing – but remember that even small amounts can have a dramatic effect when your memory is already struggling.

Try to write your own list below of ways that help *you* to cope.

1 _____

2 _____

3 _____

4 _____

5 _____

Negative thoughts

We all have negative thoughts. For example, one might be "If I have to talk to someone, then I won't be able to know what to say". These thoughts are not always realistic and are rarely helpful. Often, worries about what other people will think of them mean that people with dementia do less and spend more time in their home. This, in turn, means that they feel

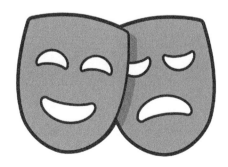

even worse. Discussing these worries with people close to you can help you to find more positive ways of thinking, such as "If I forget a word, then people won't mind".

Relaxation exercises

During the session, there will be the chance to practice one or more forms of relaxation together as a group. Try to find a way to continue to practice this every day at home.

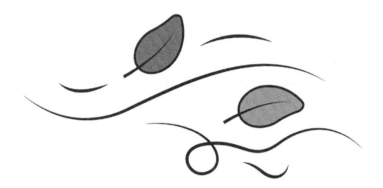

WEEK FOUR HANDOUT: FINDING A WAY THROUGH FEELINGS

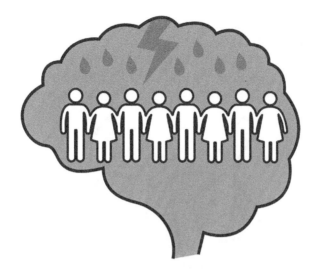

How does dementia make you feel?

- Forgetting things can make people feel anxious or stressed.
- Some people have said that dementia makes them feel angry, frustrated, sad, frightened about the future, anxious, embarrassed or stupid.
- Can you remember what you felt like when you were first told about your dementia?
- Were you

  - Angry about how unfair it was?
  - Depressed at the news?
  - Anxious about the future?
  - Relieved to have an answer?

- How have you felt since then?
- Have you felt

  - Embarrassed when you forget something?
  - Frustrated at your memory?
  - Worried about the future?
  - Guilty when other people help you?

Ups and downs

Most people have times when they are down as well as up. Sadness is a normal reaction to life's struggles, setbacks and disappointments. Many people use the word "depression" to explain these kinds of feelings, but depression is much more than just sadness.

There are lots of different ways that people cope with depression:

- Some people may deny having any problems and will play things down.
- Other people may use distractions, so will keep themselves busy to avoid feeling bad.
- Some people find it useful to talk to people for support.
- There are also people who make a joke out of it to try to cope better.

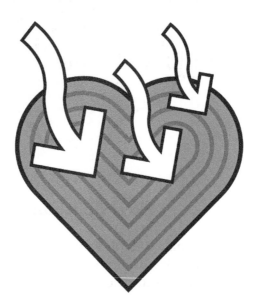

Losing confidence

There is no "right or wrong" way to cope with feelings. However, one trap that it's important to avoid is that it is easy to put off doing things if you're worried about making a mistake.

Often, this leads on to people losing confidence and then gradually giving up more and more.

Breathing and relaxation exercises

In last week's group, we tried some relaxation exercises. Remember to continue to practice these – they will help you to manage your stress!

WEEK FIVE HANDOUT: RELATIONSHIPS – TO TELL OR NOT TO TELL?

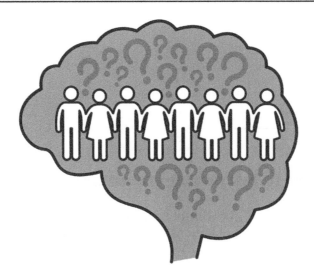

Reactions of strangers

Often, people who have dementia worry that if other people find out about the diagnosis, then they will not want to know them, or will reject them in some way. Because of this, they may decide not to tell anyone and become very self-conscious when they're out in case they make a mistake.

However, in general, most people are either too busy getting on with life to notice, or would be sympathetic rather than rejecting.

Often, the biggest problem is that people cope with their dementia by staying at home or avoiding situations that might be upsetting for them. As well as having to deal with the memory problems that the dementia causes them, they also now have to avoid situations where other people might notice there is something wrong. This, in turn, adds to the problems that we've been discussing in the last few weeks.

The advantages and disadvantages of telling other people about your illness

Take a moment to list the advantages and disadvantages of sharing your illness with others.

Advantages	Disadvantages

Would you want to tell people about having dementia?

Who would you feel you can talk to about having dementia? How would you like to tell them? Feel free to talk this through with your partner or family.

Who would you want to tell?	How would you want to tell them?

Coping with social situations

When you have a problem with your memory, the people around you may be keen to help, but may not know how to do this. It can be useful to think how you would like people to help you.

Here are some common examples of how people say they like to be helped:

People sometimes like

✓ Being given a suggestion if they can't remember a word.
✓ Being given a prompt.
✓ Having plenty of time to remember.
✓ Others joking *with* them (not at them).
✓ Getting help when they ask for it.
✓ Other people being sympathetic.
✓ People writing things down for them.
✓ Being tactfully reminded.
✓ Talking to one or at most two people at a time.

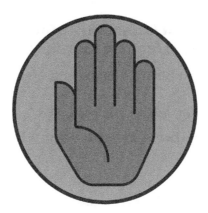

People don't like

☹ Having it pointed out to them when they repeat themselves.
☹ Being given too much information to take in.
☹ Being interrupted so they lose their thread.
☹ Having others jump in too soon without giving them time to work it out.
☹ Being rushed.
☹ Others speaking too quickly.
☹ Being in large group conversations.
☹ Having others take over and giving help when it isn't necessary.
☹ Others being impatient.
☹ Being put on the spot by questions like "What have you done today?"

Helping others to help you

In general terms, there are three golden rules:

✓ **Explain your situation.** For instance, you might tell people you have a problem, for instance, "My memory is not very good these days", so that they can understand and make allowances for you.
✓ **Be clear about what you want.** For instance, let people know if you would rather do things yourself so that they don't take over, or ask people to slow down if they are rushing you.
✓ **Show appreciation when help is given.** When people are helpful, make sure that you thank them. If you do need help, ask in a nice way.

Discuss with your family or friends what you find helpful and what you don't. It might be useful to write a list together as a reminder. This will help you both decide what you need to do more of and what you need to do less of.

Some examples of ways of asking for help

✓ **Being put on the spot/asked for information (for instance, telephone number, reference number)**

  ➢ Tell people that you have a memory problem and explain you need some extra time.
  ➢ Ask if you can come back/ring back later.

✓ **Seeing the doctor and remembering what to ask/what was said**

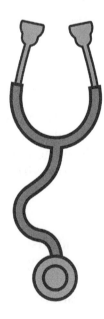

- ➢ Write questions down before you go.
- ➢ Write down what is said at the time or while it is fresh in your mind.
- ➢ Remember that it can be helpful to have someone with you.

✓ **Being criticised**

- ➢ Spend time talking to the person and explaining how you feel.
- ➢ Ask the person to stop doing it/suggest an alternative that they might say so that you don't feel criticised.
- ➢ Remember that they might not mean anything by it/nobody's perfect.

✓ **People jumping in/assuming you can't remember or do something**.

- ➢ Find a way of telling them that you *can* do it or would like to do it.

Explain that sometimes you might not be able to remember something immediately but with a little more time you might be able to.

WEEK SIX HANDOUT: WHAT IS DEMENTIA?

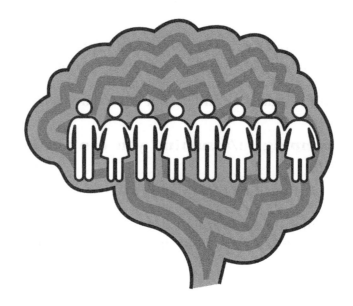

Different forms of dementia

It is important to remember that different people are affected by dementia differently. However, most people with dementia may experience some or all of the following symptoms:

- **Memory loss,** particularly of recent events. This may not be severe at first, but it is likely to become progressively worse.
- Problems **finding the right words** for what you want to say.
- Feeling **disoriented.** For example, not recognising familiar streets and becoming confused about the time of day.
- Having trouble **thinking clearly** and **doing practical tasks** that you used to do easily.
- Problems with **mobility** or **balance** or **visual perception**.
- **Changes in behaviour** – but this may be a reaction to the dementia such as sense of insecurity.

The two main forms of dementia are:

Alzheimer's disease

What is Alzheimer's disease? This is caused by damage to the nerve cells in the brain. The pattern of damage can vary between individuals, so that the difficulties experienced by one person will not be exactly the same as the next.

What causes Alzheimer's disease? Although there are many theories as to why Alzheimer's disease happens, we still don't really know what causes it, other than that it is more common with age.

Is it something that can be passed on to my children? There is an inherited form of the disease, but this is rare. Only in a very small number of highly unusual cases, which occur early in life, is Alzheimer's disease passed from one generation to the next.

Is there any treatment? There is no cure for Alzheimer's disease. However, some people are able to have some medication that can help with some of the problems of a poor memory. The most common of these is called Aricept.

Does it become worse? Alzheimer's disease is a progressive illness, but the speed at which Alzheimer's disease gets worse varies. Current research is looking at whether staying active and living healthily may help to slow this down.

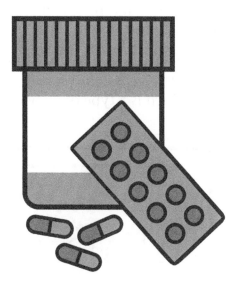

Vascular dementia

What is vascular dementia? This is caused by blockages or bleeding within the brain. This is often linked with heart disease and has the same risk factors – such as high blood pressure and high levels of cholesterol.

Can vascular dementia be passed on? This can happen, but only in the way that risks for heart disease in general can be passed on. Recent research suggests that the factors that make vascular dementia more likely are also risk factors of Alzheimer's disease.

Is there any treatment? There are no cures for vascular dementia, but you can try to reduce the risk of this becoming worse:

✓ Make sure you keep your blood pressure under control.
✓ If you smoke, then try to stop or cut down.

✓ If you drink alcohol, then make sure you drink in moderation.
✓ If you are a diabetic, then make sure you keep this under control.
✓ Make sure you take a good amount of exercise.
✓ Eat a healthful diet.
✓ Maintain social contact and hobbies as far as possible.

Who can help me?

- **Your GP.** When you first recognised that you had problems with your memory, you may have gone to see your GP. They may have asked about your medical history and done blood and urine tests to rule out the possibility of other conditions that could cause similar symptoms.
- **Memory clinics.** Your GP will probably have referred you to a specialist doctor or assessment centre for more detailed tests. This will have helped to determine what type of dementia you have so that you can receive the best type of treatment. They may also have requested a head scan to be done.
- **Head scan.** If, after the GP examination and the memory tests, it is still unclear about what type of dementia someone has, they may be sent for a head scan, which is a type of x-ray of the brain.

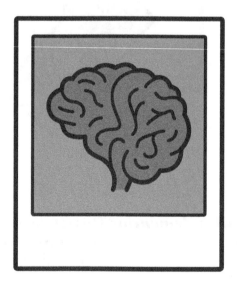

- **Memory assessments.** Either your GP or the memory clinic will almost certainly have carried out a memory test with you. One that is often used to help find out if someone has dementia is the "Mini-Mental State Examination (MMSE)". In this test, the GP will ask some questions and test attention and ability to remember words. How people score in this sort of test indicates how serious their condition is.

WEEK SEVEN HANDOUT: LIVING AS WELL AS YOU CAN

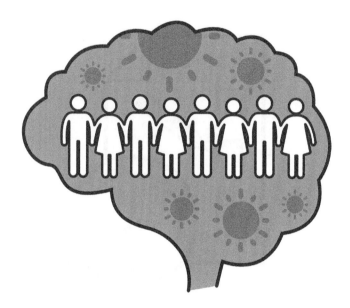

In the last session, we discussed how dementia is sometimes described as a "journey". This implies that you still have some way to go on the journey – and that it is important to think about how you can live as well as you can. For example, James McKillop, who became an advocate for the rights of people living with dementia after he was diagnosed, wrote:

> *Being told I had dementia was like a door re-opening after a difficult time in my life – new challenges, new opportunities. . . . I want people to under-stand that dementia isn't an end, it's a new beginning where you do things differently. While some things change forever there is a lot you still can do.*

Often, people find it hard to think about the future because they know that their problems will become worse. In today's session, we will briefly describe ways in which you can think about the future and prepare for it by making decisions now.

Taking charge of your life

Not everybody wants to think about these things, but some people find it helpful to feel that they have made decisions about their future. Often, this is something that a person can do, and then forget about – safe in the knowledge that if things become worse, then they have made preparations. Amongst the ways in which you could take charge of your life are:

- ✓ Talking to people around you about the future
- ✓ Making a lasting power of attorney
- ✓ Making a will
- ✓ Making a "living will" (advance decisions and advance statements)

Lasting power of attorney and advance statements

A lasting powers of attorney (LPA) is one of a number of ways to plan ahead. Other ways to plan ahead are advance statements or advance decisions. These allow you to put in writing that you want to refuse certain treatments, or your preferences about other care choices.

An LPA lets you choose a person you trust to act for you if you come to a point where you can't make decisions yourself. This person is referred to as your "attorney", and you can choose what decisions they are allowed to make for you.

One type of LPA covers decisions about your property and finances, while the other covers decisions about your health and welfare. You can choose to designate both types or just one. You can appoint the same person to be make decisions for both, or you can have different attorneys.

If you want to create an LPA, then there are forms you need to complete before they are registered – these are available on the internet, or the Alzheimer's Society can provide you with information about this.

Other things you might think about are putting your finances in order and making a will, or updating a will you have already made.

Driving

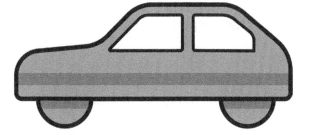

Having a diagnosis of dementia is not in itself necessarily a reason to stop driving. What matters, from both a legal and a practical point of view, is whether you are still able to drive safely.

However, if you have been given a diagnosis of dementia and you want to continue to drive, then you must, by law, inform the Driver and Vehicle Licensing Agency (DVLA).

The DVLA will send you a questionnaire for your permission for them to contact your GP and/or specialists. On the basis of the information they get back, they will make a decision as to whether you can continue to drive. They may also ask you to take a driving test.

You must also immediately inform your car insurance company. If you don't, then your policy may become invalid.

Although giving up driving is often hard, there are many ways around the problems that not driving can create – for instance, the money that you save will often more than cover the cost of getting a taxi more regularly.

What alternatives do you have to driving a car?

What can you do to change your situation?

Is there anything that you can do to help you to feel better?

- ✓ Taking things up that you haven't done for a while (which may perhaps need to be done in a different way)
- ✓ Picking up a hobby or attending a club
- ✓ Sharing ideas of hobbies/clubs people attend
- ✓ Thinking about doing mental exercises such as crosswords and quizzes on TV.
- ✓ Having a healthy lifestyle – getting exercise and having a good diet
- ✓ Asking yourself, how have you coped with difficult times in the past? Are there things that helped you then that you think could help you now?

What else can you do to change your situation?

WEEK EIGHT HANDOUT: STAYING ACTIVE

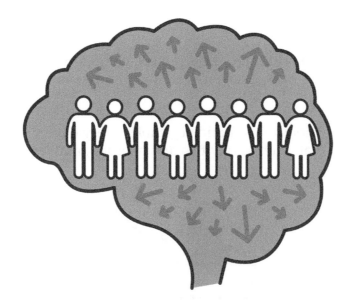

The more active we are, the less we are affected by illnesses. The evidence also suggests that having a healthier lifestyle may mean having a slightly better memory.

Physical exercise

Evidence shows that exercise helps people stay well for longer. Being physically active also helps to prevent depression and helps you feel well. You could take a short walk for 20 minutes every day, for example, walk a dog if you have one. You could also go out to play with grandchildren or exercise your upper body when sitting down.

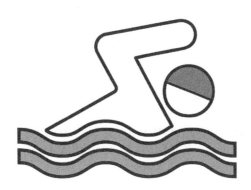

Smoking

If you smoke, then try to cut this down.

Diet and nutrition

What we eat is important for how we feel. Good food also helps the body and the brain to work efficiently, so make sure you have enough of the good stuff.

- Eat five portions of fruit and vegetables every day.
- Eat "good" fat, such as oily fish and avocado, and less "bad" fat, such as red meat.

Mental activity

Keep your brain and mind active by doing various exercises and having fun playing games. This can, in turn, help you feel more confident and able. You could, for example:

- Read the newspaper/magazines
- Work on jigsaw puzzles
- Solve crossword puzzles and sudoku
- Play card or board games with your friends or family
- Find something to do every day that you feel good at
- Find something to do every day that you enjoy

Social activity

Research shows that people who are social and have lots of contact with other people are happier. Keeping in touch with close friends and family regularly can also help your mind be active. This will, again, be beneficial to your well-being, confidence and abilities. You could, for example:

✓ Have a cup of tea or coffee with family, friends, neighbours or your church group if that is where you go
✓ Go to local support groups
✓ Go shopping and do other activities outside the home with other people
✓ Meet new people
✓ DEEP (http://dementiavoices.org.uk) provides further information and opportunities to link up with others who have dementia
✓ Contribute to research – many people like the chance to contribute to research in dementia. If you want to do this, then the Join Dementia Research Register is a good place to start (www.joindementiaresearch.nihr.ac.uk/).

Index

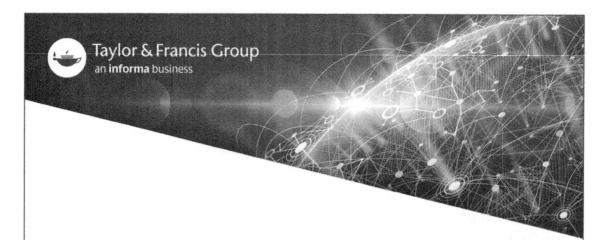
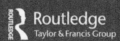
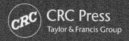

Printed and bound by CPI Group (UK) Ltd, Croydon, CR0 4YY

22/10/2024

01777638-0016